Fresh & Foraged Foods

for

Land Hermit Crabs

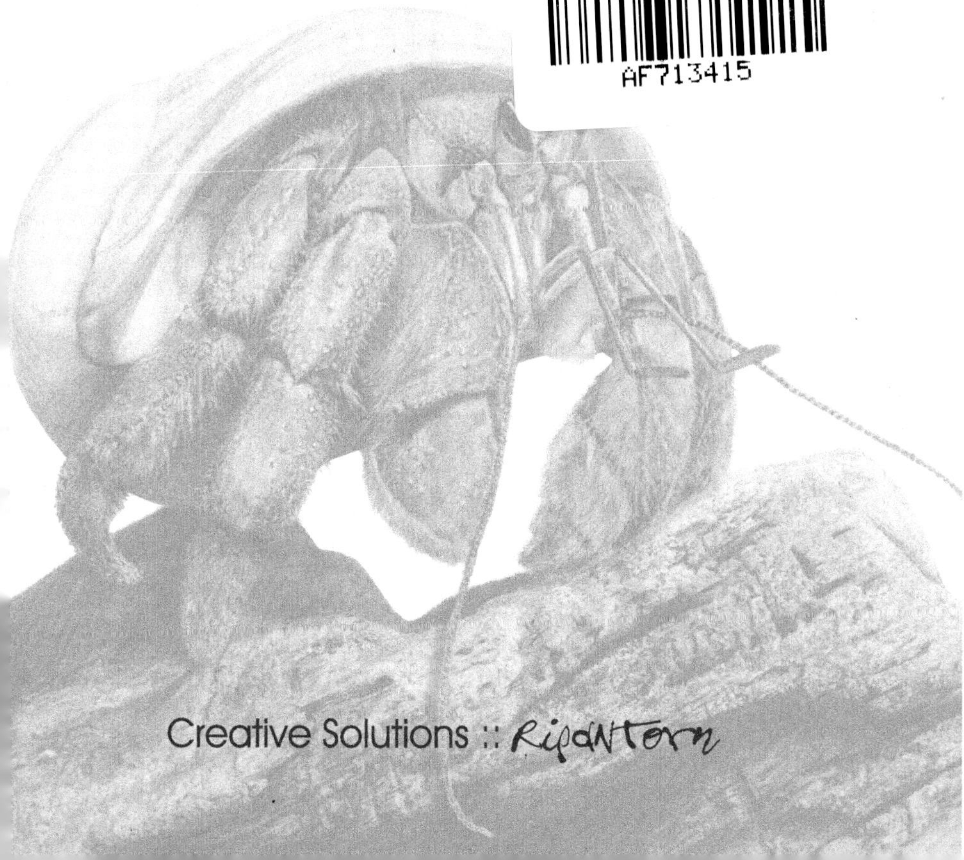

Creative Solutions :: RipNTorn

Limits of Liability & Disclaimer of Warranty:

Please do your own research. "You", the caretaker, are ultimately responsible for what you provide your land hermit crabs. In all cases with regard to any items you may choose to introduce to your crabitat:

"When in doubt - leave it out."

Content compilation, cover art
& graphic design by:

info@ripdntorn.com

This guide is available in various formats through:
MyHungryHermit. | myhungryhermit.com

ISBN: 978-1-7375423-0-8 (pocket guide, first edition)
978-1-7375423-1-5 (paperback, premium color, first edition)
978-1-7375423-3-9 (paperback, black & white, first edition)
978-1-7375423-4-6 (hardcover, first edition)

Library of Congress Cataloging-in-Publication Data is available from the author.
First printed in the United States of America.

Dedication

To Jonathan Livingston Crab and his loving and dedicated caretaker for forty-five years, Carol Ann Ormes:

May your legacy continue to inspire us all.

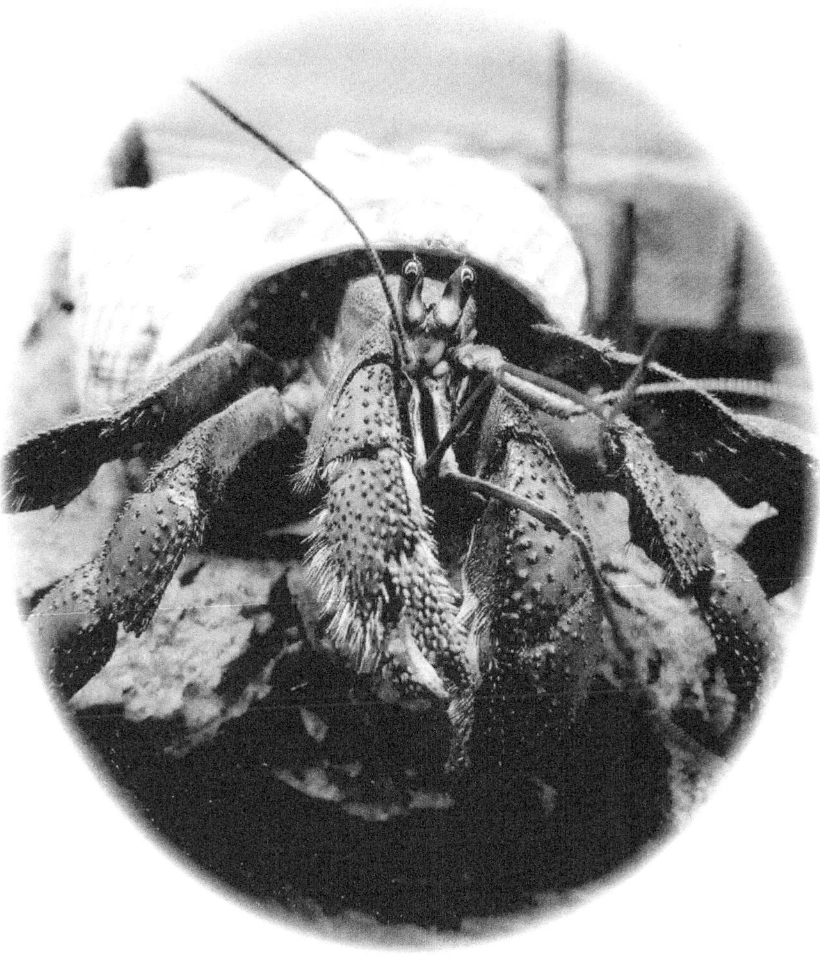

Photo Credit: Mike Vukoder, July 2019.

Jonathan Livingston Crab

(Cherished from August 1976 - February 14, 2021)

A special "Thank You" to the

Contributing Editors

Stacy Griffith, Land Hermit Crab Owners Society,
The Crab Street Journal

Complete hermit crab care guides, hermit crab food, supplements, and supplies.

lhcos.org

crabstreetjournal.org

Land Hermit Crab Owners Society (LHCOS) Group - facebook.com/groups/landhermitcrabowners

Mary Akers, Earth Water Fire Studio,
Hermit House Captive Breeding Program

Hermit crab food, supplements, and supplies.
Hermit crab related art, pottery, and feeding dishes.

maryakers.com/inthecrabitat

EarthWaterFireStudio.etsy.com

Courtney Iris Karr, BioactiveFX, Cholla Queen

Hermit crab food, supplements, & supplies.
Cholla wood, natural habitat decor, and bioactive supplies.

bioactivefx.com

BioactiveFX1.etsy.com

Amazon - Cholla Queen

Jeanne Singhass, Because of Crabs (Moss & Such)

Hermit crab food, moss, lichen, bark, wood, and other foraged items.

BecauseofCrabs.etsy.com

Foraging Group - http://bit.ly/MossSuch
(facebook.com/groups/742973182745815)

Adopt – Don't Shop!

Land Hermit Crab Owners Society (LHCOS)
Land Hermit Crab Adoption Center

Responsible rehoming and adoption program for land hermit crabs, including Hermit House captive-bred hermit crabs. Applications accepted online.

Hermits in need of homes, fosters, or transport assistance:

https://lhcos.org/adoption-program-beta/

Captive-Bred application:

http://bit.ly/CaptiveBredHCs*

Facebook:

https://www.facebook.com/HermitCrabAdoptions

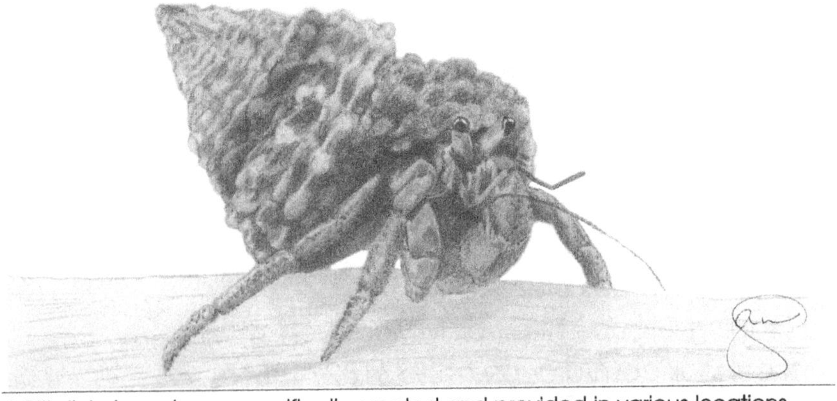

* Bitly links have been specifically created and provided in various locations throughout this publication to increase the reader's ease of access to information provided by webpages featuring long web addresses.

Table of Contents

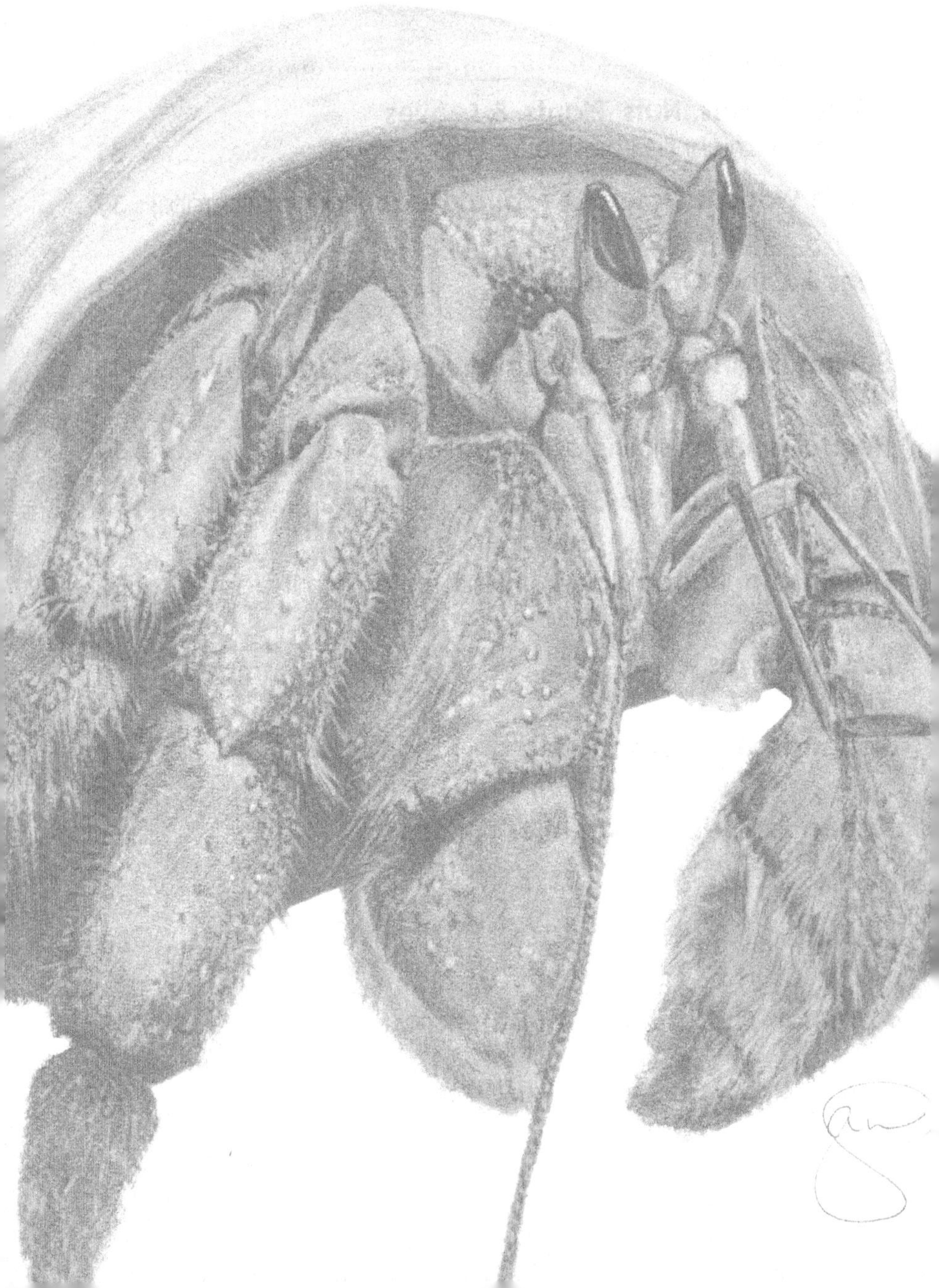

Hermit Crabs are omnivorous crustaceans and natural scavengers. They have a diverse appetite and eat a wide range of items – many of which can be found already in the refrigerator, pantry, or right outside the doorway. The following pages include some, but certainly not all, of these items.

To begin, here are a few...

General Suggestions & Guidelines

⋙ Feed foods with minimal exposure to pesticides when possible. "Organic" does not necessarily mean "free from chemicals and pesticides" – just synthetically manufactured ones. Organic farmers are permitted to use naturally sourced insecticides.[1] Because insects and hermit crabs share the same scientific classification (*Arthropoda*, invertebrates), it is possible that any substance used to repel and kill insects may affect hermit crabs in the same manner.

⋙ To remove any possible organic and synthetic pesticide residue, wash and scrub all fresh fruits and vegetables thoroughly.[1]

⋙ Washing may not entirely remove chemicals from flowers, leaves, branches, or bark. It is best to forage in known untreated areas.[1]

⋙ Do not use flowers or plants recently acquired from a florist or nursery as they have likely been treated with pesticides not rated for food consumption.

⋙ Avoid chemicals, iodized table salt, and plants that are typically toxic to other animals, especially invertebrates.[4] There is little formal research with regard to plant toxicity and hermit crabs, so it is best to err on the side of caution.

⋙ Steer clear of preservatives and artificial ingredients in commercial human, pet, fish, and hermit crab foods (see "Bad Additives").

⋙ Use seasonings deemed safe for hermit crabs when cooking foods. Avoid offering leftover foods with unknown seasoning content and items containing the generic word "seasonings". The term "unseasoned", when used in this guide, indicates that any additional spices should be reviewed for safety before offering – or left unseasoned.

⋙ Dark, leafy greens should be cooked as many contain high, soluble oxalates – molecules that bind to calcium, preventing its absorption by the body. Boiling (most effective) or steaming any vegetable considered high in oxalates can help break down the compound. Many foods high in oxalates contain other nutritional benefits, so, rather than eliminating the foods entirely, consider feeding them in moderation as part of a varied diet.[2]

⋙ All shellfish should be baked, boiled, or steamed. Raw and undercooked seafood, such as clams, mussels, oysters, and scallops, harbor bacteria (*Vibrio parahaemolyticus, Vibrio* species)[3] and have been known to cause bacterial disease and tailrot in shrimp and marine crustaceans.[5]

⋙ Providing a constant source of calcium, like cuttlebone, calcium carbonate, and/or crushed oyster shells within the crabitat can help ensure your crabs have access to the calcium that they need.

In addition, greensand and organic worm castings are also recommended to be kept in the crabitat at all times, as they provide natural nutrients, trace elements, and minerals.

⋙ Because hermit crabs are scavengers and liable to taste anything, things that aren't typically food have also been included amongst the relevant lists (i.e. wood for climbing, decorative pods for hiding, aquatic plants in water, living bioactive cleanup crew insects). They aren't necessarily a part of a diet, but their potential toxicity is relevant when they are introduced to a hermit crab's environment.

⋙ The intention of this guide is not to address living plants in a crabitat, including aquatic plants in filtered water bowls. However, it should be noted that – whether purchased or foraged – all live plants should be quarantined and/or sterilized prior to introduction. It is the reader's responsibility to conduct this additional and necessary research.

Everything else in the following "safe for hermit crabs" list may be served raw, cooked, freeze-dried, or dehydrated (unsulphured, without preservatives) unless otherwise noted.

Pages that would otherwise be blank have been formatted for note taking and additions throughout.

Items deemed "unsafe", "unpopular", or "unknown" have been printed with a gray background in an effort to minimize errors made in haste.

While every precaution has been taken to provide accurate and authoritative information regarding foods for land hermit crabs, "you", the caretaker, are ultimately responsible for what you provide your land hermit crabs. In all cases with regard to any items you may choose to introduce to your crabitat:

"When in doubt - leave it out."

Helpful Symbols

found within this section:

The lack of a food-related symbol in no way diminishes the nutrient content available in that item or the added benefits of offering variety in a diet.

♥ - highlights typically popular and favorite foods, though in no way indicates the only foods that should be offered.

Ca - signifies items that are high in calcium.

§ - identifies foods high in protein. Varied animal and plant proteins should be offered daily and comprise 50% of the diet.

✲ - denotes items with carotenoids and flavonoids, beneficial color boosting pigments that occur naturally.

✹ - symbolizes items that should be cooked, baked, boiled, or steamed to reduce or eliminate oxalates, plant-based toxins, bacteria, & parasites. Plants with this symbol should be fed in moderation as part of a varied diet.

❦ - indicates an item (or its parts like wood or bark) that isn't primarily food, but may be aesthetically pleasing as crabitat decor or used for environmental enrichment (i.e. wood for climbing, decorative pods for hiding, natural shells for food dishes, aquatic plants in water, living bioactive cleanup crew insects). This does not mean it will not get munched on...

---

[1] Griffith, Stacy. "Organic Explained."
[2] Spritzler, Franziska. "Oxalate (Oxalic Acid): Good or Bad?"
[3] Oregon Health Authority. "Safe Eating of Shellfish."
[4] The Crabstreet Journal. "FAQ What foods are good and bad for hermit crabs?"
[5] Biomin. "Vibrio in shrimp aquaculture."

Foods Generally Accepted As Safe
(for hermit crabs)

Acacia (*Acacia senegal*, *A. seyal*, gum, wood)

Açaí (*Euterpe oleracea*, fruit, hearts of palm, leaves)

Acer / Maple (flowers, leaves - not *Acer rubrum*, baked/ steamed seed, wood)

Acerola (*Malpighia emarginata*, Barbados Cherry, fruit only)

Acorn (*Quercus*, crushed)

Acorn Caps

Acorn Squash (*Cucurbita pepo* var. *turbinata*, vegetable, seed, pulp, blossoms)

Adzuki Beans (*Vigna angularis*)

African Violet Flowers (*Saintpaulia* species)

Agave (*Agave americana, A. deserti,* flowers, stalks, do not confuse with *Agave lechuguilla*)

Air Plants (*Tillandsia*, Bromeliad family)

Alaria (*Alaria longicruris, A. esculenta,* seaweed)

Alder (*Alnus glutinosa, A. incana,* European/Common/Black, Grey Alder, dried cones, wood)

Alfalfa (*Medicago sativa*, hay, sprouts)

Algae (see specific varieties in this category)

Alligator (meat, bones, marrow)

Almond (*Prunus dulcis*, shelled nut, raw, roasted, unsalted, unseasoned, no leaves or wood)

Almond Butter (all natural, no sugar, salt, corn syrup, hydrogenated oils, or xylitol) ♥

Amaranth

Amla Fruit (*Phyllanthus emblica*, Indian Gooseberry)

Anacharis (*Elodea*, aquatic plant)

Anchovy (meat, bones, skin, eyes; if canned, no preservatives or added salt) S

Anchovy Oil (small drop or mixed with food)

Antlers (Deer, Elk, Moose, etc., natural, untreated) Ca ❦

Apple (*Malus* genus, fruit only, no seeds) ♥ ✨

Apple Sauce (unsweetened, no additives) ✨

Apricot (*Prunus armeniaca*, fruit only, no pits) ✨

Aprium / Apriplum (*Prunus aprium*, plum/apricot hybrid, Pluots, Plumcots, fruit only, no pits) ✨

Arame (*Eisenia bicyclis*, kelp) ✨

Arbutus (*Arbutus unedo,* Strawberry Tree, fruit, wood) ❦

Aronia Berry (*Rosaceae* family, Chokeberry, fruit only, do not confuse with "chokecherries" from *Prunus virginiana*) ✨

Artemia and Eggs (*Artemia nauplii*, Brine Shrimp) S ✨

Artichoke (*Cynara cardunculus* var. *scolymus*, Globe Artichoke, flower, inner petals, heart, stem, not marinated) S

Ash (*Fraxinus*, bark, wood) ❦

Asian Pear (*Pyrus pyrifolia*, fruit only, no seeds)

Asparagus (*Asparagus officinalis*) S ✨ ✿

Aspen (*Populus*, leaves, bark, wood) ❦

Astaxanthin (naturally sourced from *Haematococcus pluvialis*, *Xanthophyllomyces dendrorhous*, etc.) ✨

Azomite

Baby Food (most organic types, check ingredients)

Bacacuia Gourd (dried, natural, untreated) ❦

Badderlocks (*Alaria esculenta*, seaweed) Ca S ✨

Bael Tree Pods (*Aegle marmelos*, Bell Cup, dried, natural, untreated) ❦

Bald Cypress Wood (*Taxodium distichum,* Swamp Cypress) ❦

♥- popular | Ca - calcium | S - protein | ✨ - color enhancing | ✿ - cooked | ❦ - habitat enrichment

Banana (*Musa* genus, fruit, leaves, no peel) ♥ ✨

Banana Leaves (*Musa* genus) ❦

Barbados Cherry (*Malpighia emarginata*, fruit only) ✨

Barley (*Hordeum vulgare*) ĉa

Barley Grass (*Hordeum vulgare*) ✨

Bass (meat, bones, skin, eyes) §

Basswood Leaves (*Tilia*)

Bat Guano (heat sterilized)

Beach Grass (*Ammophila, Psamma* P. Beauv.)

Beans / Legumes (*Fabaceae* family) ĉa § ✹

Bee Balm Flowers (*Monarda*)

Bee Pollen ♥

Beech (*Fagus grandifolia*, leaves, nuts, bark, wood) ❦

Beechnuts (*Fagus grandifolia*, feed raw sparingly) ✹

Beef (meat, organs, bones, marrow, horns, feces) ♥§

Beetle Grubs / Larvae (freeze-dried, frozen, canned) §

Beets (*Beta vulgaris*, root, greens, high in oxalates) ✨ ✹

Bell Cup (*Aegle marmelos*, Bael Tree Pod, dried, natural, untreated) ❦

Bell Pepper (*Capsicum*, all color varieties, no stems, leaves, or plant) ✨

Bellani Balls / Pods (*Aegle marmelos*, dried, natural, untreated, polished, not dyed) ❦

Bellflowers (*Campanula*, flowers, leaves, plant) ✨

Bent Grass (*Ammophila*, *Psamma* P. Beauv.)

Bilberry (*Vaccinium myrtillus*, fruit, blossoms) ✨

Birch, River (*Betula nigra*, leaves, bark, wood) ❦

Birch, White (*Betula papyrifera*, leaves, bark, wood) ❦

Birdhouse Gourd (*Lagenaria siceraria*, dried, natural, untreated) ❦

Bison (meat, organs, bones, marrow, horns, feces) S

Black Currant (*Ribes nigrum*, fruit only) ⁂

Black Locust (*Robinia pseudoacacia*, flowers only)

Black Raspberry (*Rubus occidentalis*, fruit, leaves) ⁂

Blackberry (*Rubus*, fruit, leaves) ⁂

Blackstrap Molasses (unsulphured, small drop or mixed with food as an occasional treat) Ca

Bladderwrack (*Gracilaria changgi*, *Fucus vesiculosis*, seaweed) Ca S ⁂

Bloodworms (dehydrated, freeze-dried, frozen) ♥ S

Blue Butterfly Pea Flowers (*Clitoria ternatea*) ⁂

Blue Spirulina (*Arthrospira*, Phycocyanin) S ⁂

Blueberry (*Vaccinium* genus, *Cyanococcus*, fruit, blossoms) ♥ ⁂

Boar (meat, organs, bones, marrow, tusks, feces) S

Bok Choy (*Brassica rapa*) ✿

Bone (cooked, raw) Ca ❦

Bone Marrow ♥ S

Bone Meal (responsibly sourced, human and domestic pet food grade) Ca

Borage (*Borago officinalis*, flowers only) ⁂

Brazil Nut (*Bertholletia excelsa*, nut meat only, feed sparingly, very high in selenium) S

Brewer's Yeast (*Saccharomyces cerevisiae*)

Brine Shrimp and Eggs (*Artemia nauplii*) S ⁂

Broccoli (*Brassica oleracea*, florets, trunk, leaves) Ca S ✿

Brown Algae (*Ecklonia cava*) S ⁂

♥- popular | Ca - calcium | S- protein | ⁂- color enhancing | ✿- cooked | ❦-habitat enrichment

Brown Rice (pre-rinsed/pre-washed) ✿

Brussels Sprouts (*Brassica oleracea*, sprouts, leaves) Ca $ ✿

Buckwheat Groats (*Fagopyrum esculentum*) $

Buddha Nut Pods (*Pterygota Alata*, dried, natural, untreated)

Burning Bush (*Euonymus alatus*, berries, leaves - red and green, wood) ♥

Butterfly Bush (*Buddleja davidii*, flowers, leaves, wood)

Butternut Squash (*Cucurbita moschata*, vegetable, seed, pulp, blossoms)

Cabbage (*Brassica oleracea*) ✿

Cacho Pods (dried, natural, untreated)

Caja Fruit (*Spondias mombin*, fruit, leaves)

Calcium Carbonate Powder Ca

Calci-worms (dehydrated, freeze-dried, canned) Ca $

Calendula Flowers (Marigold)

California Wild Rose Flowers (*Rosa californica*)

Camellia (*Camellia japonica*, flowers only)

Camu Camu Fruit (*Myrciaria dubia*, fresh, powdered)

Cantaloupe (fruit flesh, seed, pulp, blossoms, no rind)

Caribou (meat, organs, bones, marrow, antlers, feces) $

Carnation (*Dianthus caryophyllus*, flowers only)

Carrots (all color varieties, root, well washed leaves)

Cashew ("raw", roasted, unsalted, unseasoned) $

Cashew Apple (*Anacardium occidentale*, fruit only; the seed, a cashew, requires additional preparation)

Cashew Butter (all natural, no sugar, salt, corn syrup, hydrogenated oils, or xylitol) ♥ $

Catappa Leaves (*Terminalia catappa*, Indian Almond) ♥

Catfish (meat, bones, skin, eyes) $

Cattle Blood (responsibly sourced, dried, powdered) $

Cattle Bone (responsibly sourced) ĉa

Cauliflower (*Brassica oleracea*, florets, trunk, leaves) ĉa $ ✿

Caviar (check any added ingredients) $

Cayenne Pepper (*Capsicum annuum*, no stems, leaves, or plant) ⁂

Celery Leaves (*Apium graveolens*)

Centipedes (dead, freeze-dried) $

Chamomile Flowers (*Matricaria chamomilla*) ⁂

Chard (*Beta vulgaris*) ✿

Cherimoya (*Annona cherimola*, fruit only, no seeds)

Cherry (*Prunus avium*, fruit only, no pits) ⁂

Chestnuts (for human consumption, genus *Castanea*) $

Chia (*Salvia hispanica*, seeds, sprouts) ♥$

Chicken (meat, organs, bones, feet, feathers, eggs) $ ✿

Chickpeas (*Cicer arietinum*, Garbanzo Bean) ĉa ✿

Chickweed (*Stellaria media*, flowers, leaves, plant)

Chile Pepper (*Capsicum annuum*, no stems, leaves, or plant) ⁂

Chinese Bayberry Fruit (*Morella rubra*) ⁂

Chlorella (*Chlorella vulgaris*, algae) $ ⁂

Chokeberry (*Aronia*, *Rosaceae* family, fruit only, do not confuse with "chokecherries" from *Prunus virginiana*) ⁂

Cholla Wood (*Cylindropuntia*, "Choya", natural, unpainted) ❦

Chondracanthus Chamissoi (red algae) $ ⁂

Cicada Exoskeletons $

Cilantro (*Coriandrum sativum*)

♥- popular | ĉa - calcium | $- protein | ⁂- color enhancing | ✿- cooked | ❦-habitat enrichment

Cipó Escada Wood (*Bauhinia* genus, dried, natural, untreated)

Clams (meat, untreated shell - whole or crushed)

Cockroaches (feeder variety, dead, freeze-dried)

Coconut (*Cocos nucifera*, meat, husk, shell, water)

Coconut Flour

Coconut Oil (small drop or mixed with food)

Coconut Palm (*Cocos nucifera*, leaves, nut, heart, wood)

Cod (meat, bones, skin, eyes)

Cod Liver Oil (small drop or mixed with food)

Collard Greens (fresh or cooked, low in oxalates)

Copepods

Coral (untreated)

Coralline (*Lithothamnium calcareum*, red algae)

Coreopsis (Tickseed, flowers, leaves, stems)

Coriander (*Coriandrum sativum*)

Cork Bark (*Quercus suber*)

Corn (*Zea mays*, all color varieties, vegetable, cob, corn silk, inner husk layers, kernels - whole or ground, fresh, dried, cooked)

Cornflower (*Centaurea cyanus*, flowers only)

Cornmeal

Cottonseed (*Gossypium hirsutum*)

Cottonwood (*Populus*, leaves, bark, wood)

Couscous

Crab (Blue, Dungeness, King, Rock, Snow, etc., meat, exoskeleton, not imitation, research wild caught species, not *Xanthidaes*)

Crabapple (*Malus sylvestris*, fruit only, no seeds)

Cranberry (*Vaccinium macrocarpon*, fruit, blossoms; if dehydrated, unsulphured, no additives) ⁂

Crape/Crepe Myrtle (*Lagerstroemia indica*, flowers, leaves, wood) ❦

Crayfish/Crawdads/Crawfish (meat, exoskeleton) ĉa $ ✿

Crickets (freeze-dried, frozen, canned) $

Cucumber (*Cucumis sativus*)

Cupuaçu Fruit (*Theobroma grandiflorum*) ⁂

Currants (*Ribes*) ⁂

Cuttlebone / Cuttlefish Bone (whole or powdered) ♥ ĉa

Cyclops Copepods $ ⁂

Dabberlocks (*Alaria esculenta*, seaweed) ĉa $ ⁂

Dandelion (*Taraxacum officinale*, flowers, leaves, root, do not confuse with Flatweed or other imitators) ĉa ⁂

Daphnia $ ⁂

Dates (unsulphured) ĉa

Deadnettle (*Lamium pupureum*, flowers, leaves)

Deer (meat, organs, bones, marrow, feces) $

Dogwood (*Cornus florida*, fruit, flowers, leaves, wood) ❦

Dragonfruit (*Hylocereus*) ⁂

Dubia Roaches (dead, freeze-dried) $

Duck (meat, organs, bones, feet, feathers, eggs) $ ✿

Duckweed (*Lemnoideae*, aquatic plant) ❦

Dulse (*Palmaria palmata*, seaweed) ĉa $ ⁂

Dumontia Contorta (algae) $ ⁂

Dunaliella Salina (algae) $ ⁂

Dungeness Crab (meat, exoskeleton) ♥ ĉa $ ✿

Earthworms (collected away from pesticides, dehydrated, freeze-dried, frozen, canned) §

Edamame (Soybean) §✹

Eel §✹

Egg (Chicken, Duck, Ostrich, Quail, any fowl) ♥§⁂✹

Egg Shells ôa

Eggplant (*Solanum melongena*, fruit only, no stem, leaves, or plant) ⁂✹

Elderberry Flowers (*Sambucus canadensis*) ⁂

Elk (meat, organs, bones, marrow, antlers, feces) §

Elm (*Ulmus*, hardwood varieties only, wood, bark, leaves) ❦

Emu (meat, organs, bones, feet, feathers, eggs) §✹

Escargot (unseasoned) §

Evening Primrose (*Oenothera biennis*, buds, flowers, young leaves) ⁂

False Cypress Wood (*Taxodium distichum*) ❦

Feathers (wild or from unmedicated domestic fowl) §

Feeder Bugs and Frass (Dubia, Mealworms, etc.) §

Figs (*Ficus carica* L.) ôa

Filberts (*Corylus avellana*, Hazelnuts, nut meat only, raw, roasted, unsalted, unseasoned) §

Fish (all human and domestic pet food grade species, meat, bones, skin, head, eyes, eggs; if canned, no preservatives or added salt) §

Fish Oil (small drop or mixed with food)

Flax (*Linum usitatissimum*, Linseed, sprouts, oil, seeds - crushed or whole, small amounts in moderation) §

Flaxseed Oil (small drop or mixed with food, Infrequently)

Flounder (meat, bones, skin, eyes) §

Flowering Quince (*Chaenomeles speciosa*, flowers, fruit)

Forget-Me-Nots (*Myosotis* genus)

Forsythia (*Forsythia Vahl*, Golden Bells, flowers, wood) ⁂

Freekeh (Farik, roasted green wheat) **S**

Freshwater Shrimp (dehydrated, freeze-dried) **S** ⁂

Frog Legs (human grade only, meat, bones, fresh, frozen) **S**

Frogs Mouth Pods (dried, natural, untreated) ❦

Game, Wild (meat, organs, bones, horns/antlers, feces) **S**

Gammarus Shrimp ♥ **S** ⁂

Garbanzo Beans (*Cicer arietinum*, Chickpeas) ĉα **S** ✿

Giant Kelp (*Macrocystis pyrifera*) ĉα

Gladiolus Flowers (*Gladiolus* genus) ⁂

Glasswort (*Salicornia*, stems, leaves, no seeds)

Goat (meat, organs, bones, marrow, horns, feces) **S**

Goji Berry (*Lycium barbarum, L. ruthenicum*) ⁂

Goose (meat, organs, bones, feet, feathers, eggs) **S** ✿

Gooseberry (*Ribes uva-crispa*, fruit only, no leaves, stems, or plant) ⁂

Gourds (*Cucurbitaceae* family, dried, natural, untreated) ❦

Gracilaria Gracilis (red algae) **S** ⁂

Grapes (*Vitis vinifera* species, fruit, leaves, root, vine) ♥ ⁂

Grapevine (*Vitaceae, Vitis*, leaves, root, vine) ❦

Grasshoppers (dead, freeze-dried, frozen, canned) **S**

Green Beans (*Phaseolus vulgaris*) ĉα

Green Leaf Lettuce (*Lactuca sativa*)

Green Lipped Mussel (*Perna canaliculus*) **S** ✿

Green Peas (*Pisum sativum*) **S**

♥ - popular | ĉα - calcium | **S** - protein | ⁂ - color enhancing | ✿ - cooked | ❦ - habitat enrichment

Green Seaweed (*Ulva lactuca*) ĉa S ✨

Green Tripe (from any ruminant species) S

Greensand ♥

Guano (Seabird, Bat, etc., heat sterilized)

Guava (*Psidium guajava*) ✨

Habanero Pepper (*Capsicum annuum*, no stems, leaves, or plant) ✨

Haddock (meat, bones, skin, eyes) S

Haematococcus Pluvialis (algae) S ✨

Halibut (meat, bones, skin, eyes) S

Hazel (*Corylus avellana*, leaves, nuts, bark, wood) ❦

Hazelnuts (*Corylus avellana*, Filberts, nut meat only, raw, roasted, unsalted, unseasoned) S

Hemp Hearts and Seeds (*Cannabis sativa*) S

Henbit (*Lamium aplexicaule*, flowers, leaves)

Herb Flowers (the flowering blooms only, unless otherwise listed, of anise, basil, bee balm, chives, coriander/cilantro, dill, fennel, garlic, oregano, rosemary, sage, and thyme)

Herring (meat, bones, skin, eyes; if canned, no preservatives or added salt) S

Hibiscus (*Hibiscus rosa-sinensis, H. syriacus*, flowers, leaves)

Hickory (*Carya*, leaves, shelled nuts, bark, wood) ❦

Hollyhock Flowers (*Alcea rosea*) ✨

Honey (pure, single ingredient, tiny drop or mixed with food)

Honeybush Leaves (*Cyclopia intermedia*, sold as "tea")

Honeydew (fruit flesh, seeds, pulp, blossoms, no rind) ✨

Honeysuckle (*Lonicera* species, flowers only) ✨

Horn (Cattle, Goat, etc., natural, untreated) ĉa ❦

Horn Melon (Kiwano, Jelly Melon, fruit flesh, seed, pulp, no rind)

Hornbeam (*Carpinus betulus*, leaves, bark, wood)

Hornworms (feeders only, never wild caught) *S*

Hornwort (*Ceratophyllum demersum*, aquatic plant)

Hot Peppers (*Capsicum annuum*, all varieties, no stems, leaves, or plant)

Huckleberry (*Vaccinium ovatum*, fruit, blossoms)

Hydrilla Verticillata (fresh, powdered, aquatic plant) ca

Impatiens Flowers (*Impatiens wallerana*)

Indian Almond Leaves (*Terminalia catappa*, Catappa) ♥

Indian Gooseberry (*Phyllanthus emblica*, fruit only)

Irish Moss (*Chondrus crispus*, sea vegetable)

Isopods (Pillbugs, Woodlice, Roly-polies) *S*

Jacaranda (*Jacaranda cuspidifolia, J. mimosifolia*, flowers, pods - dried, natural, untreated)

Jalapeño Pepper (*Capsicum annuum*, no stems, leaves, or plant)

Japanese Red Maple (*Acer palmatum*, leaves, wood)

Jasmine (*Jasminum officinale* only, flowers only)

Java Moss (*Vesicularia dubyana*, aquatic plant)

Jewelweed Flowers (*Impatiens capensis*, Wild Impatiens)

Jicama (*Pachyrhizus erosus*, root only, no skin, stem, seeds, or leaves)

Johnny-Jump-Up Flowers (*Viola tricolor*, *Viola* genus)

Kale (fresh or cooked, low in oxalates) ca *S*

Kangaroo (meat, organs, bones, marrow) *S*

Kañiwa (*Chenopodium pallidicaule*) ca *S*

♥- popular | ca - calcium | *S*- protein | - color enhancing | - cooked | - habitat enrichment

Katydids (dead, dehydrated, freeze-dried)

Kelp (*Laminariales*) Ca

Khorasan Wheat (*Triticum turanicum*, Kamut) $

Kiwi Fruit (*Actinidia deliciosa*) ✨

Kombu (*Laminaria Japonica*, kelp) Ca

Krill (frozen, freeze-dried, oil) ♥$

Kudzu (*Pueraria montana*, flowers, leaves, root, vine) ❦

Lamb (meat, organs, bones, marrow, horns, feces) $

Lamium (flowers, leaves)

Laverbread (*Porphyra dioica*, *P. purpurea*, seaweed) Ca $ ✨

Legumes / Beans (*Fabaceae* family) Ca $ ☼

Lettuce, Green and Red Leaf (*Lactuca sativa*)

Lichen (see Appendix B) ❦

Lilac (*Syringa vulgaris*, flowers, leaves, wood) ❦

Lingonberry (*Vaccinium vitis-idaea*, fruit, blossoms) ✨

Live Sand ❦

Liver (Poultry, Beef, Pork, etc., organ meat) $

Lobster (meat, exoskeleton) Ca $ ☼

Locusts (freeze-dried, frozen, canned) $

Lotus (*Nelumbo nucifera*, seeds, flowers, leaves, stem, root)

Lotus Seed Pods (*Nelumbo nucifera*, dried, natural, untreated) ❦

Macadamia Nuts (raw, roasted, unsalted, unseasoned) $

Mackeral (meat, bones, skin, eyes; if canned, no preservatives or added salt) $

Magnolia Flowers (*Magnolia grandiflora*)

Mandarin Orange (*Citrus reticulata*, fruit segments) ✨

Mango (*Mangifera indica*, fruit only, no seed) ♥✨

Mangosteen Fruit (*Garcinia mangostana*) ⁂

Mangrove (*Rhizophora mangle*, leaves, wood) ❦

Manure (see "Bugs & Other Odd Snacks")

Manzanita (*Arctostaphylos manzanita*, leaves, wood) ❦

Maple (*Acer*, flowers, leaves - not *Acer rubrum*, baked/ steamed seed, wood) ❦

Maple Syrup (pure, single ingredient, tiny drop or mixed with food as an occasional treat, no corn syrup) ĉa

Marigold Flowers (*Calendula*) ⁂

Marimo (*Aegagropila linnaei*, Moss Ball, aquatic plant) ❦

Marionberry (*Rubus* L. subgenus *Rubus*, fruit only) ⁂

Marram Grass (*Ammophila, Psamma* P. Beauv.)

Mealworms $

Meat (Poultry, Beef, Pork, etc., meat, organs, bones, fat) $

Melon (fruit flesh, seed, pulp, blossoms, no rind) ⁂

Mice ("Pinkies", sold frozen as reptile food) ♥$

Milk Thistle Flowers (*Silybum marianum*)

Millet (includes puffed variety, sprouts) ♥$

Mimosa Tree (*Albizia julibrissin*, Persian Silk Tree, flowers, leaves, no seed pods)

Minnows (fresh, freeze-dried, dehydrated) $

Mint (not peppermint)

Mojaban (*Sargassum fulvellum*, seaweed) ĉa $ ⁂

Molasses, Blackstrap (unsulphured, small drop or mixed with food as an occasional treat) ĉa

Mollusks (meat, untreated shell - whole or crushed) ĉa ✿ ❦

Monkey Pods/Pots (*Lecythis pisonis*, dried, natural, untreated) ❦

Moose (meat, organs, bones, marrow, antlers, feces) $

♥- popular | ĉa - calcium | $- protein | ⁂- color enhancing | ✿- cooked | ❦-habitat enrichment

Mopani Wood (*Colophospermum mopane*) ❦

Moss (fresh, dried, not preserved or dyed, see Appendix A) ❦

Mulberry (*Morus nigra, M. rubra*, fruit only) ⁂

Muscadine Grape (*Vitis rotundifolia*, fruit, leaves, root, vine) ♥ ⁂

Mushrooms (any for human consumption) S

Mussels (meat, untreated shell - whole or crushed) Ca ✹ ❦

Mustard Greens (fresh or cooked, low in oxalates) S Ca ⁂

Mysis Shrimp S ⁂

Nannochloropsis (algae) S ⁂

Nasturtium Flowers (*Tropaeolum majus*) ⁂

NatuRose (*Haematococcus pluvialis*, algae) S ⁂

Nectacot (nectarine/apricot hybrid, fruit only, no pits) ⁂

Nectarine (*Prunus persica*, fruit only, no pits) ⁂

Nereocystis (kelp) Ca

Nettle Leaves (*Urtica*, wilted, blanched, dried)

Noni Fruit (*Morinda citrifolia*) ⁂

Nopales (*Nopal cacti*, flowers, cacti) ⁂

Nori (*Pyropia* genus, *Porphyra* species, seaweed) Ca S ⁂

Nutritional Yeast (*Saccharomyces cerevisiae*)

Oak (*Quercus*, leaves, acorns, bark, wood) ❦

Oats / Oatmeal (*Avena sativa*) ♥ S

Octopus S

Offal (variety organ meats) S

Oil (Coconut, Flax, Olive, Fish, Krill, Salmon, Sunflower, unrefined, cold pressed, extra virgin, small drop or mixed with food, <u>not</u> Canola Oil)

Oil Palm Fruit (*Elaeis guineensis*)

Okra (*Abelmoschus esculentus*, high in oxalates) ĉa ☼

Olive Oil (extra virgin, small drop or mixed with food)

Oranges (*Citrus sinensis*, fruit segments) ✶✶

Orchid (*Orchidaceae*, flowers, plant) ✶✶

Ostrich (meat, organs, bones, feet, feathers, eggs) $ ☼

Owl Pellets (heat sterilized, baked)

Oxtail (meat, bone, marrow) $

Oyster $ ☼

Oyster Shells (whole, crushed) ♥ ĉa ❦

Pacific Kelp (*Macrocystis pyrifera*) ĉa

Palm Blut ❦

Palm Caps ❦

Pampas Grass (*Cortaderia selloana*)

Pansy (*Viola X Wittrockiana*, flowers, leaves) ✶✶

Papaya / Papaw (*Carica papaya*, fruit, no seeds) ♥ ✶✶

Parsley (*Petroselinum crispum*, high in oxalates) ĉa ✶✶ ☼

Parsnips (*Pastinaca sativa*, root, well washed leaves)

Partridge (meat, organs, bones, feet, feathers, eggs) $ ☼

Passionfruit (*Passiflora*, ripe fruit only, no leaves) ✶✶

Peach (*Prunus persica*, fruit only, no pits) ✶✶

Peacotum (peach/apricot/plum hybrid, fruit only, no pits) ✶✶

Peanut Butter (all natural, no sugar, salt, corn syrup, hydrogenated oils, or xylitol) ♥ $

Peanuts and Shells (boiled, roasted, unsalted, unseasoned) $

Pear (*Pyrus*, fruit only, no seeds) ✶✶

Peas (*Pisum sativum*, Green, Snow, Sugar Snap, etc., shelled, unshelled, raw or cooked) $

♥ - popular | ĉa - calcium | $ - protein | ✶✶ - color enhancing | ☼ - cooked | ❦ - habitat enrichment

Pecan (*Carya illinoinensis*, shelled nuts, bark, wood) § ❦

Peppers, Bell (*Capsicum*, all color varieties, no stems, leaves, or plant) ⁂

Peppers, Hot (*Capsicum annum*, no stems, leaves, or plant) ⁂

Persimmon (if dehydrated, unsulphured, no additives) ⁂

Petunia (flowers only) ⁂

Pfaffia Yeast (*Phaffia rhodozyma*) ⁂

Pheasant (meat, organs, bones, feet, feathers, eggs) § ✪

Phlox (*Phlox* genus, flowers, leaves) ⁂

Phoenix Worms (dehydrated, freeze-dried, canned) §

Pig (meat, organs, bones, marrow) §

Pine Nuts §

Pineapple (*Ananas comosus*) ♥ ⁂

Pink Pitaya Fruit (*Hylocereus*) ⁂

Pistachios (shelled, raw, roasted, unsalted, unseasoned) §

Plankton §

Plantain (*Musa* genus, "cooking banana", fruit, no peel) ✪

Plum (*Prunus domestica*, fruit only, no pits) ⁂

Plumcots / Pluots (*Prunus aprium*, plum/apricot hybrid, Aprium, Apriplum, fruit only, no pits) ⁂

Pomegranate (*Punica granatum*, seeds only, no root, stem, or peel) ⁂

Popcorn (popped, unpopped, whole or ground, unsalted, unseasoned, unflavored) ♥

Poplar (*Populus*, leaves, bark, wood) ❦

Pork (meat, organs, bones, marrow) §

Potato (*Solanum tuberosum*, root vegetable/tuber only, no leaves, plant, sprouts/eyes, or green potatoes)

Potato, Sweet (*Ipomoea batatas*, high in oxalates) ⁂ ✿

Poultry (meat, organs, bones, feet, feathers, eggs) § ✿

Prickly Pear (*Nopal cacti*, flowers, cacti) ⁂

Prunes (no pits, unsulphured) ĉa

Psyllium Husks

Puffed Rice

Pumpkin (*Cucurbita pepo*, seeds/pepitas, meat, pulp, blossoms, stems, leaves) ⁂

Purple Sweet Potato (*Ipomoea batatas*) ⁂

Purslane (*Portulaca oleracea*, high in oxalates) ✿

Quail (meat, organs, bones, feet, feathers, eggs) § ✿

Quinoa (pre-rinsed/pre-washed) ĉa §

Rabbit (meat, organs, bones, marrow, feces from wild or unmedicated pets) §

Raisins (unsulphured)

Rams Head / Ram's Horn Pods (*Borassus flabellifer*) ❦

Raspberry (*Rubus idaeus*, fruit, leaves) ⁂

Raspberry Leaves (*Rubus idaeus*, high in B vitamins, vitamin C, and many trace minerals, often sold as "tea") ⁂

Red Algae (*G. parvispora, G. gracilis, Chondracanthus Chamissoi*, Coralline, *Lithothamnium Calcareum*) § ⁂

Red Bud/Redbud (*Cercis canadensis* L., flowers, buds, young pods) ⁂

Red Leaf Lettuce (*Lactuca sativa*)

Rhubarb Stems (*Rheum rhaponticum*, high in oxalates, no leaves) ✿

Rice (*Oryza sativa*, pre-rinsed/pre-washed) ✿

Rice, Puffed

♥ - popular | ĉa - calcium | § - protein | ⁂ - color enhancing | ✿ - cooked | ❦ - habitat enrichment

River Birch (*Betula nigra*, leaves, bark, wood) ❦

River Shrimp (dehydrated, freeze-dried) § ⁂

Roaches (Feeder Cockroaches, Dubia, etc., dehydrated, freeze-dried, frozen, canned) §

Rodents (Beaver, Pinkies/Mice, Muskrat, etc., meat, organs, bones, marrow) §

Rolled Oats ♥§

Rooibos (*Aspalathus linearis*, often sold as "tea") ⁂

Rose (*Rosa* genus, leaves, buds, petals, hips) ⁂

Rose of Sharon Flowers (*Hibiscus syriacus*, not St. John's Wort/ *Hypericum* which shares common name) ⁂

Rotifers / Rotifera §

Royal Jelly (organic, tiny drop or mixed with food)

Rye (*Secale cereale*, seeds/berries/grain) §

Sacred Water Lotus (*Nelumbo nucifera*, flowers, leaves, seeds, seed pod, stem, root)

Sacred Water Lotus Seed Pod (*Nelumbo nucifera*) ❦

Safflower Seeds §

Sage Flowers (*Salvia officinalis*)

Salicornia (Glasswort, stems, leaves, no seeds)

Salmon (meat, bones, skin, eyes; if canned, no preservatives or added salt) § ⁂

Sand Dollars (untreated) ca ❦

Sapa / Sapucaia Pods (dried, natural, untreated) ❦

Sardines (meat, bones, skin, eyes; if canned, no preservatives or added salt) §

Sargassum Muticum (seaweed) ca § ⁂

Scallops (meat, untreated shell - whole or crushed) ca ✹ ❦

Sea Biscuits (untreated) ca

Sea Buckthorn Fruit (*Hippophae rhamnoides*) ✨

Sea Cucumber (*Holothuroidea*) $

Sea Fan, Black (*Iciligorgia schrammi*, untreated) ❦

Sea Fan, Red (*Gorgonia adamsi*, untreated) ❦

Sea Grape (*Coccoloba uvifera*, berries, leaves, wood) ❦

Sea Grasses (*Posidoniaceae, Zosteraceae, Hydrocharitaceae, Cymodoceaceae*)

Sea Palm (*Nereocystis*, kelp) ĉa

Sea Salt (no anti-caking agents)

Sea Shells (untreated, whole, crushed) ĉa ❦

Sea Sponge (untreated, not for use in water dishes) ❦

Sea Urchin (human grade meat, untreated shells & spines) ĉa ✿ ❦

Sea Whip (*Nereocystis*, kelp) ĉa

Seaberries (*Hippophae rhamnoides*, Sea Buckthorn Fruit) ✨

Seasonings, Safe (chili powder, crushed red pepper, herbs as individually listed, paprika, sea salt, turmeric, check ingredients for preservatives, additives, and/or anti-caking agents, see "Bad Additives")

Seaweed (see specific varieties in this category) ĉa $ ✨

Serrated Wrack (*Fucus serratus*, seaweed) ĉa $ ✨

Sesame Seeds (crushed or whole, paste, butter) $

Shellfish (human and domestic pet grade species, meat, untreated shell - whole or crushed) ĉa $ ✿ ❦

Shrimp (meat, exoskeleton) ♥ ĉa $ ✨ ✿

Silkworm Pupae $

Silversides (meat, bones, skin, eyes) $

Skulls (natural, untreated) ĉa ❦

Snails (human grade only, not wild caught, meat, untreated shell - whole or crushed) ĉa $ ❦

♥- popular | ĉa - calcium | $- protein | ✨- color enhancing | ✿- cooked | ❦-habitat enrichment

Snake Shed / Skin (from wild in untreated areas or unmedicated domestic pets, freeze for 48 hours)

Snow Peas (*Pisum sativum*)

Soldier Fly Larvae (dehydrated, freeze-dried, canned)

Sora Pods (*Sororoca Penca*)

Sorghum Grain (*Poaceae* family)

Soursop Fruit (*Annona muricata*)

Soybeans (Edamame)

Spaghetti Squash (*Cucurbita pepo*, vegetable, seed, pulp, blossoms)

Spanish Moss (*Tillandsia Usneoides*, not preserved or dyed)

Speedwell (*Veronica persica*, flowers, leaves)

Sphagnum Moss (*Sphagnum cymbilifolium*, not preserved or dyed)

Spider Plant (*Chlorophytum comosum*, as decor)

Spiders (non-venomous, dead, dehydrated, freeze-dried)

Spinach (*Spinacia oleracea*)

Spiralled Wrack (*Fucus spiralis*, seaweed)

Spirulina (*Arthrospira,* algae/beneficial cyanobacteria)

Spongeweed (*Codium tomentosum*, seaweed)

Springtails

Sprouts (Alfalfa, Bean, Chia, Flax, Millet, Mung Bean, Pea, bacteria susceptible - wash well or cook)

Squash (*Cucurbita pepo,* vegetable, seed, pulp, blossoms)

Squid

Squirrel (meat, organs, bones, marrow)

Star Pods / Star Anise Pods (*Illicium verum, I. anisatum*, dried pods only, no fruit)

Starfish (untreated) ĉa ❦

Starfruit (*Averrhoa carambola*, fruit, flowers, leaves; fruit is high in oxalates, feed sparingly or cook)

Strawberry (*Fragaria*, fruit, tops, young leaves) ✶

Strawberry Tree (*Arbutus unedo*, fruit, wood) ❦

Sugar Cane (*Saccharum officinarum*)

Sugarwrack (*Laminaria saccharina*, kelp) ĉa

Summer Squash (*Cucurbita pepo*, vegetable, seeds, leaves, blossoms) ✶

Sunflower (*Helianthus*, seeds, flowers, leaves) $ ✶

Sunflower Oil (small drop or mixed with food)

Sunflower Seeds (raw, roasted, unsalted, unseasoned) $

Superworms (freeze-dried, frozen, canned) $

Swamp Cypress Wood (*Taxodium distichum*, Bald Cypress) ❦

Sweet Gum Tree Pods (*Liquidambar styraciflua*, dried) ❦

Sweet Potato (*Ipomoea batatas*, high in oxalates) ✶ ✹

Swiss Chard (*Beta vulgaris*) $ ✹

Sycamore Wood (*Platanus occidentalis*) ❦

Tahini (Sesame Seed Paste, single ingredient) $

Talami Pods (*Borassus flabellifer*, dried, natural, untreated) ❦

Tamarack Blossoms (*Tamarix*)

Tangerine (*Citrus tangerina*, *C. reticulata*, fruit segments) ✶

Tart Cherry (*Prunus cerasus*, fruit only, no pits) ✶

Teak Leaves (*Tectona grandis*)

Teff (*Eragrostis tef*, fresh, grain)

Tickseed (*Coreopsis* genus, flowers, leaves, stems) ✶

Tigela Pods ❦

♥- popular | ĉa - calcium | $- protein | ✶- color enhancing | ✹- cooked | ❦-habitat enrichment

Tilapia (meat, bones, skin, eyes)

Tillandsia (Bromeliad family, Air Plants)

Timothy (*Phleum pratense*, grass, hay)

Tomato (*Solanum lycopersicum*, ripe fruit only, no leaves, stems, or plant)

Tripe (from any ruminant species)

Trout (meat, bones, skin, eyes)

Trumpet Pods (*Cariniana savu*)

Tubifex Worms (freeze-dried, dehydrated)

Tuna (meat, bones, skin, eyes; if canned, no added salt)

Turkey (meat, organs, bones, feet, feathers, eggs)

Turmeric (*Curcuma longa*)

Turnip (*Brassica rapa*, root, well washed leaves)

Venison (meat, organs, bones, marrow, antlers, feces)

Violet / Viola Flowers (*Viola* genus)

Virginia Spring Beauty (*Claytonia virginica*, flowers, plant)

Wakame (*Undaria Pinnatifida*, seaweed)

Walnuts, English (*Juglans regia*, nut meat only, raw, roasted, unsalted, unseasoned)

Water Fleas

Water Flies

Watercress (*Nasturtium officinale*)

Watermelon (fruit flesh, seed, pulp, blossoms, no rind)

Wax Worms

Wheat (*Triticum* genus, *T. aestivum, T. durum, T. turanicum*)

Wheat Germ

Wheat Grass/Wheatgrass (*Triticum aestivum*)

Whitefish (meat, bones, skin, eyes) §

Wild Boar (meat, organs, bones, marrow, tusks, feces) §

Wild Game (meat, organs, bones, marrow, horns/antlers/tusks, feces) §

Wild Impatiens Flowers (*Impatiens capensis*) ✨

Wild Petunia Flowers (*Ruellia humilis*) ✨

Wild Rice §✿

Winter Squash (*Cucurbita pepo*, vegetable, seeds, pulp, blossoms) ✨

Worm Castings (organic) ♥

Yeast, Brewer's (*Saccharomyces cerevisiae*)

Yeast, Nutritional (*Saccharomyces cerevisiae*)

Yeast, Pfaffia (*Phaffia rhodozyma*) ✨

Yellow Squash (*Cucurbita pepo*, vegetable, seeds, leaves, blossoms) ✨

Yucca (*Yucca* genus, flowers, fruit, stem, no roots or leaves)

Yumberry (*Morella rubra*) ✨

Zucchini (*Cucurbita pepo* var. *cylindrica*, Courgette, vegetable, seeds, leaves, blossoms) ✨

Notes

♥- popular | - calcium | §- protein | ✨- color enhancing | ✿- cooked | - habitat enrichment

Foraged Finds

⋙ The following lists refer to items generally found in North America. Botanical names have been provided where possible.

⋙ Consider investing in a regional, photographic field guide to native plants or download an app for plant identification to assist in identifying species. Do not harvest anything unless you are completely positive that what you are harvesting is safe for hermit crabs.[6]

⋙ Foraging should be done in remote locations like woods or at home if organic gardening is practiced. Public parks may use chemicals to keep bugs and weeds away.[6]

⋙ Never forage in an area with known or possible pesticide, insecticide, and/or herbicide use.[6]

⋙ Harvest in small amounts so that plants can regrow and repopulate with minimal damage.[6]

⋙ For your own protection, be wary of wildlife and poisonous plants while foraging.[6]

⋙ Do not trespass. Be sure that the land is not protected and make sure you have a right to harvest as some nature trails have plants that are not allowed to be destroyed or removed.[6]

⋙ Do not use flowers or plants from florists, nurseries, or garden centers as they have likely been treated with pesticides not intended for food consumption.[7] Whether purchased or foraged – all live plants should be quarantined and/or sterilized prior to introduction.

⋙ Foraged items found by the side of the road are not recommended. Highly poisonous herbicides are often used to control weeds and plants bordering roadways.[7] The proximity to pollution and roadway runoff is cause for concern.

⋙ All harvested items should be washed with dechlorinated water and live plants should be quarantined to prevent the introduction of unwanted insects/eggs into the crabitat.

⋙ Wood can be frozen, boiled, microwaved, and/or baked to eliminate unwanted pests.

⋙ Moss can be frozen without killing it in order to eliminate pests (a suggested minimum of 48 hours).

⋙ Flowers and leaves can be served fresh, air dried, dehydrated, freeze-dried, or previously frozen.[7]

⋙ Harvested plants may be kept in a container with water to keep them fresh for up to one week.[6]

---

[6] Kilamanjaro's Hermits. "Harvesting."

[7] Crab, Julia. "Safe Edible Flowers for Hermit Crabs."

Safe Flowers, Nuts, Plants, & Leaves

(that you might find outside for hermit crabs)

Acer (flowers, leaves - not *Acer rubrum*, baked/steamed seed, wood)

Acorns (*Quercus*, crushed nut, caps)

Air Plants (*Tillandsia*, Bromeliad family)

Alder (*Alnus* genus, dried cones, wood)

Alfalfa (*Medicago sativa*)

Arbutus (*Arbutus unedo*, Strawberry Tree, fruit, wood)

Aronia (*Rosaceae* family, fruit only, do not confuse with "chokecherries" from *Prunus virginiana*)

Barley Grass (*Hordeum vulgare*)

Basswood Leaves (*Tilia*)

Beach Grass (*Ammophila, Psamma* P. Beauv.)

Bee Balm Flowers (*Monarda*)

Beech (*Fagus grandifolia*, leaves, nuts, bark, wood)

Beechnuts (*Fagus grandifolia*)

Bellflowers (*Campanula*, flowers, leaves, plant)

Bent Grass (*Ammophila, Psamma* P. Beauv.)

Bilberry (*Vaccinium myrtillus*, fruit, blossoms)

Birch, River (*Betula nigra*, leaves, bark, wood)

Birch, White (*Betula papyrifera*, leaves, bark, wood)

Black Currant (*Ribes nigrum*, fruit only)

Black Locust (*Robinia pseudoacacia*, flowers only)

Black Raspberry (*Rubus occidentalis*, fruit, leaves)

Blackberry (*Rubus*, fruit, leaves)

Blue Butterfly Pea Flowers (*Clitoria ternatea*)

Blueberry (*Cyanococcus*, fruit, blossoms)

Borage (*Borago officinalis*, flowers only)

Burning Bush (*Euonymus alatus,* berries, leaves - red and green, wood)

Butterfly Bush (*Buddleja davidii*, flowers, wood)

Calendula Flowers (*Calendula officinalis*, Marigold)

California Wild Rose Flowers (*Rosa californica*)

Camellia (*Camellia japonica*, flowers only)

Chamomile Flowers (*Matricaria recutita*)

Chestnuts (for human consumption, genus *Castanea*)

Chickweed (*Stellaria media*, flowers, leaves, plant)

Chokeberry (*Aronia*, *Rosaceae* family, fruit only, do not confuse with "chokecherries" from *Prunus virginiana*)

Coconut Palm (*Cocos nucifera*, leaves, nut, heart, wood)

Coreopsis (Tickseed, flowers, leaves, stems)

Cornflower (*Centaurea cyanus*, flowers only)

Cottonwood (*Populus*, leaves, bark, wood)

Crabapple (*Malus sylvestris*, fruit only, no seeds, stems, leaves, or wood)

Crape/Crepe Myrtle (*Lagerstroemia indica*, flowers, leaves, wood)

Currants (*Ribes*)

Dandelion (*Taraxacum officinale*, flowers, leaves, root, do not confuse with Flatweed or other imitators)

Deadnettle (*Lamium pupureum*, flowers, leaves)

Dogwood (*Cornus florida*, fruit, flowers, leaves, wood)

Elderberry Flowers (*Sambucus canadensis*)

Elm (*Ulmus*, hardwood varieties only, wood, bark, leaves)

Evening Primrose (*Oenothera biennis*, buds, flowers, young leaves)

Flowering Quince (*Chaenomeles speciosa*, flowers, fruit)

Forget-Me-Nots (*Myosotis* genus)

Forsythia (*Forsythia Vahl*, Golden Bells, flowers, wood)

Gladiolus Flowers (*Gladiolus* genus)

Glasswort (*Salicornia*, stems, leaves, no seeds)

Gooseberry (*Ribes uva-crispa*, fruit only, no leaves, stems, or plant)

Grape (*Vitis vinifera, Vitaceae, Vitis*, fruit, leaves, root, vine)

Hazel (*Corylus avellana*, leaves, nuts, wood)

Hazelnuts (*Corylus avellana*)

Henbit (*Lamium aplexicaule*, flowers, leaves)

Herb Flowers (the flowering blooms only, unless otherwise listed, of anise, basil, bee balm, chives, coriander/cilantro, dill, fennel, garlic, oregano, rosemary, sage, and thyme)

Hibiscus (*Hibiscus rosa-sinensis, H. syriacus*, flowers, leaves)

Hickory (*Carya*, leaves, nuts, wood)

Hollyhock Flowers (*Alcea rosea*)

Honeysuckle (*Lonicera* species, flowers only)

Huckleberry (*Vaccinium ovatum*, fruit, blossoms)

Impatiens Flowers (*Impatiens wallerana*)

Japanese Red Maple (*Acer palmatum*, leaves, wood)

Jasmine (*Jasminum officinale* only, flowers only)

Jewelweed Flowers (*Impatiens capensis*, Wild Impatiens)

Johnny-Jump-Up Flowers (*Viola tricolor, Viola* genus)

Kudzu (*Pueraria montana*, flowers, leaves, root, vine)

Lamium (flowers, leaves)

Lichen (see Appendix B)

Lilac (*Syringa vulgaris*, flowers, leaves, wood)

Magnolia Flowers (*Magnolia grandiflora*)

Mangrove (*Rhizophora mangle*, leaves, pods, wood)

Manzanita (*Arctostaphylos manzanita*, leaves, wood)

Maple (*Acer*, flowers, leaves - not *Acer rubrum*, baked/ steamed seed, wood)

Marigold Flowers (*Calendula*)

Marionberry (*Rubus L.* subgenus *Rubus*, fruit only)

Marram Grass (*Ammophila, Psamma* P. Beauv.)

Milk Thistle Flowers (*Silybum marianum*)

Mimosa Tree (*Albizia julibrissin*, Persian Silk Tree, flowers, leaves, no seed pods)

Mint (not peppermint)

Moss (see Appendix A)

Mulberry (*Morus nigra, M. rubra*, fruit only)

Nasturtium Flowers (*Tropaeolum majus*)

Nettle Leaves (*Urtica*, wilted, blanched, dried)

Oak (*Quercus*, acorns, leaves, bark, wood)

Pampas Grass (*Cortaderia selloana*)

Pansy (*Viola X Wittrockiana*, flowers, leaves)

Pecan (*Carya illinoinensis*, nuts, bark, wood)

Petunia Flowers

Phlox (*Phlox* genus, flowers, leaves)

Poplar (*Populus*, leaves, bark, wood)

Prickly Pear (*Nopal cacti*, fruit, flowers, cactus)

Pumpkin (*Cucurbita pepo,* fruit, blossoms, leaves)

Purslane (*Portulaca oleracea*)

Raspberry (*Rubus idaeus*, fruit, leaves)

Red Bud/Redbud (*Cercis canadensis L.*, flowers, buds, young pods)

River Birch (*Betula nigra*, leaves, bark, wood)

Rose (*Rosa* genus, leaves, buds, petals, hips)

Rose of Sharon Flowers (*Hibiscus syriacus*, not St. John's Wort/ *Hypericum* which shares common name)

Sage Flowers (*Salvia officinalis*)

Salicornia (Glasswort, stems, leaves, no seeds)

Sea Grape (*Coccoloba uvifera*, berries, leaves, wood)

Sea Grasses (*Posidoniaceae, Zosteraceae, Hydrocharitaceae, Cymodoceaceae*)

Spanish Moss (*Tillandsia Usneoides*)

Speedwell (*Veronica persica*, flowers, leaves)

Squash Blossoms (*Cucurbita pepo*)

Strawberry (*Fragaria*, fruit, tops, young leaves)

Strawberry Tree (*Arbutus unedo*, fruit, wood)

Sugar Cane (*Saccharum officinarum*)

Sunflower (*Helianthus*, seeds, flowers, leaves)

Sweet Gum Tree Pods (*Liquidambar styraciflua*, dried)

Tamarack Blossoms (*Tamarix*)

Tickseed (*Coreopsis* genus, flowers, leaves, stems)

Tillandsia (Bromeliad family, Air Plants)

Timothy (*Phleum pratense*, grass, hay)

Violet / Viola Flowers (*Viola* genus)

Virginia Spring Beauty (*Claytonia virginica*, flowers, plant)

Wheat / Wheatgrass (*Triticum aestivum*)

Wild Impatiens Flowers (*Impatiens capensis*)

Wild Petunia Flowers (*Ruellia humilis*)

Yucca (*Yucca* genus, flowers, fruit, stem, no roots or leaves)

Notes

Safe Wood & Natural Crabitat Decor

(for hermit crabs)

⋙ Including wood and vines for climbing and decorative pods and shells for hiding and foraging activities enriches the environment and provides stimulation for land hermit crabs.

⋙ Foraged items can be frozen, boiled, or baked to eliminate unwanted pests. A repeated freeze/thaw/rinse method over the course of several days is instrumental in evicting hidden insects when boiling and baking is not an option.

⋙ If purchased, wood and natural decor items should be natural, untreated, unpainted, and not dyed. See "Contributing Editors" shop links.

⋙ All of the items in this category should be thoroughly dried before introduction to minimize the formation of mold within the crabitat.

Safe Wood & Vines

Acacia (*Acacia senegal, A. seyal, Mimosoideae* family)

Acer / Maples

Alder, Common (*Alnus glutinosa*, European, Black)
Alder, Grey (*Alnus incana*)

Arbutus (*Arbutus unedo*, Strawberry Tree)

Ash (*Fraxinus*)

Aspen (*Populus*)

Bald Cypress (*Taxodium distichum*, Swamp Cypress)

Beech (*Fagus grandifolia*)

Birch, River (*Betula nigra*)

Birch, White (*Betula papyrifera,* Paper Birch)

Burning Bush (*Euonymus alatus*)

Cholla (*Cylindropuntia,* "Choya")

Cipó Escada Vine (*Bauhinia* genus)

Coconut Palm (*Cocos nucifera*)

Cork Bark (*Quercus suber*)

Cottonwood (*Populus*)

Crape/Crepe Myrtle (*Lagerstroemia indica*)

Dogwood (*Cornus florida*)

Driftwood (Mangrove, Manzanita, Mopani)

Elm (*Ulmus*, hardwood vaieties only)

False Cypress (*Taxodium distichum*)

Forsythia (*Forsythia Vahl*, Golden Bells)

Grapevine and Root (*Vitaceae, Vitis*)

Hazel (*Corylus avellana*)

Hickory (*Carya*)

Hornbeam (*Carpinus betulus*)

Japanese Red Maple (*Acer palmatum)*

Kudzu Vine and Root (*Pueraria montana*)

Lilac (*Syringa vulgaris*)

Mangrove (*Rhizophora mangle*)

Manzanita (*Arctostaphylos manzanita*)

Maple (*Acer*)

Mopani (*Colophospermum mopane*)

Oak (*Quercus*)

Pecan (*Carya illinoinensis*)

Poplar (*Populus*)

Sea Grape (*Coccoloba uvifera*)

Strawberry Tree (*Arbutus unedo*)

Swamp Cypress (*Taxodium distichum*, Bald Cypress)

Sycamore (*Platanus occidentalis*)

Natural Pods & Decor

Acorn Caps

Antlers (Deer, Elk, Moose, etc.)

Bacacuia Gourd

Bael Tree Pods (*Aegle marmelos*)

Bell Cup (*Aegle marmelos*)

Bellani Pods / Balls (*Aegle marmelos*)

Birdhouse Gourd (*Lagenaria siceraria*)

Bones

Buddha Nut Pods (*Pterygota Alata*)

Cacho Pods

Coconut Shells

Coral

Frogs Mouth Pods

Gourds (*Cucurbitaceae* family, dried only)

Horns (Cattle, Deer, Goat, etc.)

Jacaranda Pods (*Jacaranda cuspidifolia*)

Lotus Seed Pods (*Nelumbo nucifera*)

Monkey Pods / Pots (*Lecythis pisonis*)

Palm Blut

Palm Caps

Rams Head / Ram's Horn Pods (*Borassus flabellifer*)

Sacred Water Lotus Seed Pods (*Nelumbo nucifera*)

Sand Dollars

Sapa / Sapucaia Pods

Sea Fans (*Iciligorgia schrammi, Gorgonia adamsi*)

Sea Shells

Sea Sponge

Sea Urchin Shells and Spines

Shells (from food sources, Clam, Mollusk, Oyster, Scallop, Snail/ Escargot, useful as food and foraging dishes)

Skulls

Sora Pods (*Sororoca Penca*)

Star Pods / Star Anise Pods (*Illicium verum, I. anisatum*)

Starfish

Sweet Gum Tree Pods (*Liquidambar styraciflua*)

Talami Pods (*Borassus flabellifer*)

Tigela Pods

Trumpet Pods (*Cariniana savu*)

Notes

Bugs & Other Odd Snacks

Hermit Crabs are scavengers and "cleaners", feasting on a variety of things found washed ashore or laying on the coastal forest floor – including bugs, dead animals, and animal excrement. Because of an increasing desire of many keepers to offer natural oddities to their animals' diets, several of the following items are also available for purchase.

Bugs

Insects are an excellent source of protein and chitin. They are generally fed to hermit crabs dead, dehydrated, freeze-dried, or canned without preservatives or added ingredients.

- Freeze canned leftovers to keep them fresh.
- Do not collect insects that may have died as the result of insecticide poisoning.

Beetle Grubs/Larvae

Calci-worms

Centipedes

Cicada Exoskeletons

Crickets

Grasshoppers

Hornworms (feeders only, never wild caught)

Isopods (Pillbugs, Woodlice, Roly-polies)

Katydids

Locusts

Mealworms

Roaches (feeder cockroaches, dubia)

Silkworm Pupae

Soldier Fly Larvae

Spiders (non-venomous species)

Superworms

Waxworms

Other Odd Snacks

Bloodworms (frozen, freeze-dried)

Cattle Blood (dried, powdered)

Earthworms (collected away from pesticides, freeze-dried, frozen, canned)

Feathers (wild or from unmedicated domestic fowl)

Feet and Necks (Chicken, Duck, Turkey, from any fowl)

Fish Eyes / Heads (fresh, frozen, freeze-dried, dehydrated)

Frog Legs (fresh, frozen, human grade only)

Green Tripe (from any ruminant species)

Offal (variety organ meats)

Owl Pellets (heat sterilized, baked)

Pinky Mice ("Pinkies", sold as frozen food for reptiles)

Snake Shed / Skin (from wild in untreated areas or unmedicated domestic pets, freeze for 48 hours)

Notes

The OTHER Other Odd Snacks

Hermit crabs can eat the feces of most animals, wild or domestic, that have a healthy, whole food diet and have not been on medication, ingested preventative dewormers/antiparasitic drugs, or been in contact with topical insecticides (i.e. domestic animals with flea and tick preventative measures in place).

⋙ Visit the "Contributing Editors" shop links for a variety of items in this category.

⋙ When foraging, be aware that parasites may shed in excrement and that it can harbor viruses, fungi, and bacteria harmful to humans. Wear gloves during collection and dry all poop outside. Foraged feces can be baked as an added precaution against harmful organisms. Commercially available products like chicken manure and bat guano are typically already heat sterilized.

Bat Guano (heat sterilized)

Chicken Manure (heat sterilized)

Cow Dung / Manure

Deer Droppings

Elk Droppings

Frass (from feeder bugs, Dubia, Mealworm, etc.)

Goat Manure

Horse Dung / Manure

Moose Droppings

Rabbit Droppings

Seabird Guano (heat sterilized)

Sheep Manure

Worm Castings

Notes

Putting it all together:

A Beginner's Banquet

What follows are a few items that represent highly nutritious options when mixed and offered with fresh foods. They provide an excellent base for creating a convenient, homemade, dehydrated crab diet.

⋙ These items can be found online, at natural food or apothecary stores, in organic or natural food sections of grocery stores, and through all-natural hermit crab food suppliers.

⋙ Stores with bulk foods may also offer several of these items by weight.

⋙ Leaf, flower, fruit, vegetable, and seed items may be foraged or purchased fresh, dehydrated, or freeze-dried.

⋙ Foraged leaves and flowers may be air dried in a dark, warm location by hanging bunches upside down or laying a single layer on a screen or parchment-lined baking sheet, tossing often.

⋙ Without an actual dehydrator, many fruits and vegetables can be dehydrated in an oven set at 140°F. This process may take several hours. Place sliced items in a single layer on baking sheets lined with parchment paper, rotating trays from top to bottom every 30 minutes.

⋙ Many of the dried leaf and flower items are often sold as a "tea." Double check the ingredients for any additives.

⋙ Other items that are beneficial to keep on hand

include coconut oil (for cooking eggs, mixing with food), greensand, and organic worm castings.

For a base diet mix, start with:

- Dandelion leaves and/or root (also sold as "tea")
- Hemp hearts/seeds (meal, ground, whole)
- Red raspberry leaves (also sold as "tea")
- Rooibos (also sold as "tea")
- Spirulina

Add a couple varieties of dried flowers:

- Calendula (also sold as "tea")
- Chamomile (also sold as "tea")
- Hibiscus (also sold as "tea")
- Rose, hips and/or petals (also sold as "tea")

Add some unsulphured, unsweetened dried fruit:

- Coconut
- Papaya
- Persimmon
- Pineapple
- Prunes and/or Raisins

Extra staple items to consider adding over time or when creating additional mixes:

- Amaranth, chia, and/or pre-rinsed quinoa
- Almonds and/or English walnuts
- Blue corn, meal or ground
- Chlorella and/or kelp powder
- Dried insects
- Pumpkin seeds and/or sunflower seeds
- Wheat germ

Serve some of your homemade mix with a variety of fresh fruit, vegetables, proteins, and other items from the "safe" list for a daily, wholesome diet!

See "Helpful Hints (for storing dried hermit crab foods)" for tips on storing your completed mix.

**"Variety's the very spice of life,
That gives it all its flavour."**

~ William Cowper, The Task (1785).

To read more about the overall nutritional needs of land hermit crabs, visit »»

http://bit.ly/CrabNutrition
https://crabstreetjournal.org/download/hermit-crab-feeding-guide/

http://bit.ly/CrabNutrition2
https://crabstreetjournal.org/download/hermit-crab-nutrition-table/

Sources:

Bonnie Plants. "How to Dry Your Harvest." https://bonnieplants.com/gardening/how-to-dry-your-harvest/ (http://bit.ly/DehydrateStuff)

Campbell, Kerie. "Going Natural Beginner's List" (2005). https://crabstreetjournal.org/blog/2015/04/07/going-natural-beginners-list/ (http://bit.ly/NaturalBeginner)

Notes

Helpful Hints

(for storing dried hermit crab foods)

It is not necessary to buy huge quantities of each ingredient used in the preparation of any homemade dry diet! Smaller, more manageable quantities may be available in all-natural hermit crab food shops, allowing a broader variety of foods at a lesser overall cost outlay. See "Contributing Editors" shop links.

Dried (dehydrated, freeze-dried) foods are not immune to environmental factors that may diminish their nutritional benefits or shorten their shelf life. Because all dried foods are susceptible to insect contamination and moisture reabsorption, it is important to properly store items purchased in larger quantities to preserve their efficacy.[8]

- Pack foods in clean, dry insect-proof containers as tightly as possible to minimize air content. Canning jars, freezer containers with tight-fitting lids, freezer bags, and vacuum packing are good options.[8]

- Pack foods in amounts that can be used all at once or in amounts that will be used in single recipes. Each time a package is opened, the food is exposed to air and moisture that can lower the quality of the food and result in spoilage.[8]

- Dried foods should be stored in cool, dry, dark areas or in the freezer. As food quality is affected by heat, the higher the temperature, the shorter the storage time.[8]

- Recommended storage times for dehydrated foods range from 4 months to 1 year.[8]

- Recommended storage times for opened freeze-dried foods range from 6 months to 1 year. With the use of oxygen absorbers, sealed product can be stored for up to 25 years! You can determine if freeze-dried food has become overexposed to moisture and oxygen if the food becomes chewy and gummy.[9]

---

[8] National Center for Home Food Preservation. "Drying."
[9] Ready Store. "What is the Shelf-Life of an Open Can?"

Notes

More helpful hints regarding

Dried Foods in the Crabitat...

⋙ Freeze-dried and dehydrated foods tend to last a little longer inside the crabitat, especially when placed closer to the heat source and farther from the water dishes.

⋙ Fresh foods typically need to be removed after 24 hours. If the fresh foods appear untouched, Stacy Griffith of the Land Hermit Crab Owners Society and *The Crab Street Journal* suggests that "because hermit crabs are scavengers and cleaners, slightly older, riper fruits and vegetables – like what might drop from a tree or vine in nature – may be more appealing."

⋙ Offering a variety of fresh and dried foods in separate dishes or in divided dishes, such as those offered in the "Contributing Editors" shops, makes changing out foods that decay faster than others a little easier.

⋙ Dried and dehydrated mixes are particularly helpful when planning a vacation feeding schedule for a pet sitter.

⋙ Many freeze-dried items are available as nutritionally dense powders. According to Courtney Iris Karr of BioactiveFX, "Freeze-dried powders have around 98% of their natural moisture removed. This process also retains more nutrients — especially the vitamins and minerals [compared to other drying processes]. However, they do tend to suck up humidity from our tanks which can make them turn gummy and begin to harden in the dish. I suggest mixing them with other, more dense, food items or sprinkling the powders on things such as popped popcorn or puffed millet."

Notes

The Unsafe, Unpopular, & Unknown
(for hermit crabs)

⋙ All items in this category have been printed on this gray background in an effort to minimize errors made in haste.

⋙ The items in this section should be avoided as some may be poisonous when eaten, used as natural insect repellents and insecticides, or lack sufficient research to make a determination regarding their effect on land hermit crabs biologically. All are considered "use at your own [crab's] risk."

⋙ Though some parts of a fruit or plant may be edible, other parts are not. For instance, while the fruit of an apricot is safe, its pit is not. Some of these items and their unsafe parts are contained in this list.

⋙ A couple of the items have been added for no reason other than they are typically unpopular. While a lemon or a lime may not be toxic, hermit crabs generally will not eat sour citrus, and therefore they have been included in this list.

⋙ Lastly, a few items in this section may simply require additional caution when identifying, foraging, or sourcing (i.e. clover, cattails).

⋙ There are many flowers and plants that are considered poisonous. Because two plants may be known by the same common name - one toxic, one edible - botanical names have been provided where possible.

⋙ Do not provide an item if there is any uncertainty in identification.

⋙ Items that are marked with a "cooked" symbol (✿) in the "Foods Generally Accepted As Safe" portion of this guide are not addressed in the following section. The symbol (✿) was offered as a way to identify items that may contain high soluble oxalates, natural plant defense compounds that can be neutralized by heat or water (see Appendix C), or bacteria/viruses/parasites that may be harmful to hermit crabs and/or the humans handling the raw items (i.e. shellfish, salmonella potential in poultry and their eggs and untreated feces). Should the reader choose to offer any of the items without first cooking them or include the plants marked with this symbol (✿) as a larger portion of a repetitious daily diet – it is considered "at your own [crab's] risk."

This portion of the guide is to create a pause before offering an item to land hermit crabs – with much of the research available being based on mammals, reptiles, amphibians, and occasionally other invertebrates.

Hermit crabs are wild animals and the challenge for any keeper of wildlife is to provide safe, nutritious foods in a captive diet while using a variety of available foods that are not necessarily from the animal's native environment. Whereas various species have developed ways of dealing with toxins present in their natural habitat and from their primary food sources (by avoidance, limiting intake, specialized adaptations, see Appendix C), if the hermit crab has not been repeatedly exposed to the same, typically toxic items in order to evolve a way to deal with them, then one might assume that items listed as "unsafe" for other species may also be unsafe for hermit crabs. At the very minimum, toxicity with regard to hermit crabs may be unknown and one must weigh the nutritional benefits possible against any potential risk factors that have been identified for other animals and invertebrates.

In short – one must ask:

> What are the actual nutritional benefits of offering an item of unknown toxicity over one generally regarded as safe?
>
> Is the novelty of presenting a potentially unsafe item worth the risk?

Helpful Symbols

found within this section:

- These ingredients are commonly added to commercial and processed foods, and should be avoided until additional research is available with regard to their effects on hermit crabs. These items are also listed in "Bad Additives."

- Items with this symbol are often used as natural insect repellents/insecticides and may also have other toxic properties. Because insects and hermit crabs share the same scientific classification (*Arthropoda*), it is possible that these items may affect hermit crabs in the same manner.

Notes

Acer rubrum - leaves (Red Maple, unidentified toxin affecting horses)

Aconite / Aconitum (*Aconitum* genus)

African Lily (*Agapanthus africanus*)

Agapanthus (*Agapanthus* genus)

Agave - raw sap, leaves (Avoid *Agave lechuguilla* in its entirety. With over 200 agave species, make sure an edible one is identified if offering the cooked flowers and stalks.)

Ageratina (*Ageratina* genus, Snakeroots)

Alder, Red or White - bark (*Alnus rubra, A. rhombifolia*, "Oregon" Alder)

Allium (*Allium* genus)

Almond, Bitter - seeds/nuts, stems, leaves, wood (*Prunus dulcis* var. *amara*)

Almond, Sweet - leaves, wood (*Prunus dulcis*)

Aloe Vera (*Aloe barbadensis*)

Amanita (Some species of the mushroom *Amanita* genus are not considered toxic, but it is safest to assume that they all are. Proper identification can be difficult.)

Amaryllis (*Hippeastrum, Amaryllidaceae* family)

Amaryllis Belladonna (*Amaryllis, Amaryllidaceae* family)

American Hellebore (*Veratrum viride*)

Amsinckia (*Amsinckia* genus, Fiddlenecks)

Anemone (*Anemone* genus, Windflowers)

Angel's Trumpets (*Brugmansia* genus)

Anise - seeds (*Pimpinella anisum*, blossoms are safe)

Anti-Caking Agents

Apple - seeds, stems, leaves, wood (*Malus* genus, use of the wood within a crabitat is controversial, repeated exposure to pesticides is likely if sourced from an orchard, additional research is necessary)

Apricot - seeds, stems, leaves, wood (*Prunus armeniaca*)

Aprium / Apriplum - seeds, stems, leaves, wood (*Prunus aprium*, hybrid of two *Prunus* species - plums and apricots, also called Pluots or Plumcots)

Artificial Color, Flavoring, and Sweeteners

Ascorbyl Palmitate

Aspartame

Aster (*Asteraceae* family)

Asteraceae Family (The Daisy family is enormous and, while there are some members that aren't considered toxic, it is safest to assume that they all are. Identification between look-alike species is difficult.)

Atropa Belladonna (Deadly Nightshade, Belladonna)

Autolyzed Yeast

Autumn Crocus (*Colchicum autumnale*)

Avocado - leaves, skin, pit, unripe flesh (*Persea americana*. Ripe flesh may be safe, but no supporting documentation exists regarding the toxin "persin" and its effects on crustaceans.)

Azalea (*Rhododendron* genus)

Bamboo - fresh, live (*Bambusoideae*, shoots contain levels of cyanide-inducing glycosides)

Baneberry (*Actaea*)

Barley Malt

Basil (*Ocimum basilicum*, source of linalool, blossoms are safe)

Bay Leaves (*Laurus nobilis*)

Beach Apple (*Hippomane mancinella*, Manchineel Tree)

Beach Pea (*Lathyrus manumus, L. japonicus*)

Begonia (*Begonia* species, *Begoniaceae* family)

- food additive | - natural insect repellent or insecticide

Benzoates

Betel Nut Palm (*Areca catechu*)

BHA (Butylated hydroxyanisole)

BHT (Butylated hydroxytoluene)

Bindweed (*Convolvulus* genus)

Birch Sugar (Xylitol)

Bird of Paradise (*Strelitzia* genus)

Birdhouse Gourd - fresh, juice (*Lagenaria siceraria*)

Bitter Almond - seeds/nuts, stems, leaves, wood (*Prunus dulcis var. amara*)

Bittersweet (*Solanum celastrus*, Nightshade family)

Black Eyed Susan (*Rudbeckia hirta, Rudbeckia fulgida,* Coneflower Rudbeckia)

Black Locust - seeds, stems, leaves, bark, wood (*Robinia pseudoacacia*)

Black Pepper (*Piper nigrum*, source of piperine)

Black Walnut (*Juglans nigra*)

Bleeding Heart (*Dicentra, Lamprocapnos spectabilis*)

Bloodroot (*Sanguinaria canadensis*)

Bluebonnet / Lupines (*Lupinus* genus)

Blue-Green Algae (*Microcystis aeruginosa*, cyanobacteria, microcystin toxin; Not all "blue-green algae" is toxic. Additional research is necessary.)

Bottlebrush - flowers (*Callistemon* genus)

Bottlebrush Buckeye (*Aesculus parviflora*)

Bougainvillea (*Bougainvillea* genus)

Bouillon

Boxwood (*Buxux sempervirens*)

Briars (possible puncture hazard)

Broth (the generic word "broth")

Brugmansia (*Brugmansia* genus, Angel's Trumpets)

Buckthorn (*Rhamnus* genus)

Buttercup (*Ranunculus* genus)

Butylated Hydroxyanisole (BHA)

Butylated Hydroxytoluene (BHT)

By Products (the generic word "by product")

Caladium

Calcium Caseinate

Calcium Silicate

Calla Lily (*Zantedeschia aethiopica*, contains insoluble calcium oxalate crystals)

Camphor Tree/Laurel (*Cinnamomum camphora*)

Cannabis (varieties with THC content)

Canola and Canola Oil (*Brassica napus*)

Capsicum - stem, leaves, plant (Nightshade family)

Carboxymethylcellulose/CMC

Cardinal Flower (*Lobelia* genus)

Carnation - leaves (*Dianthus caryophyllus*)

Carolina Jessamine (*Gelsemium sempervirens*)

Cassava - root, plant (*Manihot esculenta*)

Castor Bean (*Ricinus communis*, Castor Oil Plant)

Castor Oil

Catnip (*Nepeta cataria*)

Cat's Ear (*Hypochaeris radicata*, dandelion look-alike, toxic to horses, toxin unknown)

- food additive | - natural insect repellent or insecticide

Cattails (*Typha*. No sources indicate that the plant itself has toxic properties. However, *Typha* is very efficient at absorbing pesticides, metals, and other toxic chemicals from polluted water.[10] These are most likely stored in the rhizome and it is possible that the harmful substances absorbed could find their way into the leaves and other parts of the plant.)

Cedar - needles, wood (*Cedrus* genus)

Celandine (*Chelidonium* genus)

Cerbera Odollam (Suicide Tree)

Cherimoya - seeds (*Annona cherimola*)

Cherry - seeds, stems, leaves, wood (*Prunus avium*)

Cherry Laurel (*Prunus laurocerasus*)

Chestnut, Horse (*Aesculus hippocastanum*, all parts)

China Berry Tree (*Melia azedarach*)

Chinese Evergreen (*Aglaonema* genus, contains insoluble calcium oxalate crystals)

Chinese Lantern (*Physalis alkekengi*)

Chives (*Allium schoenoprasum*, blossoms are safe)

Chocolate

Chokecherry (*Prunus virginiana*)

Christmas Berry (*Heteromeles arbutifolia*, Toyon)

Christmas Rose (*Helleborus* genus)

Chrysanthemum Species / Mums (*Asteraceae* family, source of pyrethrum/pyrethrin)

Cinnamon

Citronella (*Cymbopogon*)

Citrus Fruit - sour, seeds, rind (Sour varieties are generally unpopular. Limonene is sourced from the rind and is especially concentrated in orange rinds. Post harvest fungicides are typically applied to non-organic citrus.[11])

Citrus Trees - leaves, wood (lemon, lime, kumquat, orange, tangerine, etc.)

Clematis (*Clematis* genus)

Clove - buds, oil (*Syzygium aromaticum*)

Clover (*Trifolium*. The red variety *Trifolium pratense* is susceptible to the fungus *Rhizoctonia / Slafractonia leguminicola* which contains the alkaloid toxins slaframine and swainsonine. Horses are highly sensitive.[12] Their effects on hermit crabs is unknown. Others like the white variety *Trifolium repens* may contain cyanide-inducing glycosides and, to further confuse the situation, the percentage of the glycosides can vary based on climate and elevation.[13] While some members of the clover genus are not subject to the same concerns, the reader should use caution in foraging/sourcing prior to introducing it to the crabitat.)

Cocoa

Coffee Grounds

Colchicum (*Colchicum* genus)

Columbine (*Aquilegia* genus)

Common Privet (*Ligustrum* genus)

Copper Sulfate

Coral Plant (*Jatropha multifida*)

Crabapple - seeds, stems, leaves, wood (*Malus sylvestris*, use of the wood within a crabitat is controversial, repeated exposure to pesticides is likely if sourced from an orchard, additional research is necessary)

Creeping Charlie (*Glechoma hederacea*)

Crocus (*Crocus* genus)

Crown of Thorns (*Euphorbia milii*)

Cubé Plant (*Lonchocarpus utilis*)

Custard Apple - young fruit, seeds, leaves, wood (*Annona reticulata*)

- food additive | - natural insect repellent or insecticide

Cyanobacteria (*Microcystis aeruginosa,* microcystin toxin. Not all cyanobacteria is toxic. Additional research is necessary.)

Cyclamen (*Cyclamen* genus, Persian Violet)

Cypress (*Cupressus* genus, *Cupressacea* family)

Daffodil (*Narcissus* genus)

Dahlia (*Dahlia* species, *Asteraceae* family, mildly toxic to dogs, cats, and horses, toxin unknown, flowers likely safe when fed in moderation with regard to tortoises, no roots)

Daisy Family (The Daisy family, *Asteraceae*, is enormous and, while there are some members that aren't considered toxic, it is safest to assume that they all are. Identification between look-alike species is difficult.)

Daphne (*Daphne* genus)

Datura (*Datura* genus, Thornapples, Jimsonweeds, Devil's Trumpets)

Daylily / Day Lily (*Hemerocallis* genus. Easily confused with the toxic *Lilium* genus. The flowers and buds of the Daylily species are likely safe in moderation, but not leaves or roots. *Hemerocallis* and *Lilium* are both highly toxic to cats.)

Deadly Nightshade (*Atropa Belladonna*)

Death Camas (*Toxicoscordion venenosum*)

Death Cap (*Amanita phalloides*)

Delphinium (*Delphinium* genus)

Derris Elliptica (*Derris elliptica* species)

Destroying Angel (*Amanita virosa*)

Devil's Ivy (*Epipremnum aureum*, contains insoluble calcium oxalate crystals)

Devil's Trumpets (*Datura* genus)

Diatomaceous Earth

Dieffenbachia (*Dieffenbachia* genus, contains insoluble calcium oxalate crystals)

Dill - seed, stem, leaves (*Anethum graveolens*, blossoms are safe)

Dittany (*Origanum dictamnus*)

Doll's Eyes (*Actaea* genus)

Dumbcane (*Dieffenbachia* genus, contains insoluble calcium oxalate crystals)

Echinacea (Coneflower, flowers and leaves are likely safe; do not confuse with *Helenium* genus, Sneezeweed, Black Eyed Susan, or other imitators)

Eggplant - stems, leaves, plant (*Solanum melongena*, Nightshade family)

Elderberry - seeds, stems, leaves, roots (*Sambucus canadensis*. The berries are likely safe, if cooked. Cooking destroys the cyanide-inducing glycosides in the seeds.)

Elephant Ear (*Colocasia* genus, Taro, contains insoluble calcium oxalate crystals)

Emulsifiers (i.e. xanthan gum, canola oil, carboxymethylcellulose/CMC, polysorbate 80/P80, microcrystalline cellulose/MCC)

English Ivy (*Hedera helix*)

Enzymes and Enzyme Modified, anything

Ethoxyquin

Eucalyptus (*Eucalyptus globulus*)

Euphorbia (*Euphorbia* genus)

European Pennyroyal (*Mentha pulegium*)

Evergreens (cedar, juniper, pine, redwood, etc.)

False Dandelion (*Hypochaeris radicata*, dandelion look-alike, toxic to horses, toxin unknown)

False Hellebore (*Veratrum* genus)

False Jasmine / Jessamine (*Gelsemium sempervirens*, *Gelsemium* genus)

- food additive | - natural insect repellent or insecticide

Feverfew (*Tanacetum parthenium*)

Fiddle Leaf Fig (*Ficus lyrate*)

Fiddlenecks (*Amsinckia* genus)

Flatweed (*Hypochaeris radicata*, dandelion look-alike, toxic to horses, toxin unknown)

Fleabane (*Erigeron* genus)

Four O'Clocks (*Mirabilis* genus)

Foxglove (*Digitalis purpurea*, *Digitalis* genus)

Fungi (in general, to include mushrooms not identified for safe human consumption, toxic species vary)

Fungus (in general, toxic species vary)

Gardenia (*Gardenia jasminoides*)

Garlic (*Allium sativum,* blossoms are safe)

Garlic Mustard (*Alliaria petiolata*)

Gelsemium (*Gelsemium* genus)

Geranium (*Pelargonium* genus)

Golden Pothos (*Epipremnum aureum*, contains insoluble calcium oxalate crystals)

Goldenrod (*Solidago Odora.* Flowers are likely safe. Leaves are toxic to sheep and susceptible to toxic fungus. Easily confused with *Haplopappus heterophyllus* [14], a plant containing trematone which is toxic to grazing animals.[15])

Gourds - fresh, juice (the typically inedible gourds of the *Cucurbitaceae* family, *Citrullus colocynthis*, *Lagenaria Siceraria*, Bottle Gourd, colocynths, ornamental gourds)

Green Hellebore (*Helleborus viridis*)

Heavenly Bamboo (*Nandina* species)

Hellebore (Helleborus genus, *Ranunculaccea* family)

Hemlock (*Conium maculatum*)

Holly (*Ilex* genus)

Honeysuckle - leaves, stems (*Lonicera* species)

Hornworms, Wild Caught (In the wild, these caterpillars feed on solanaceous plants - tomato, tobacco, and the Nightshade family. They absorb the toxins from the leaves of these plants which can potentially poison the animals that eat them. If they are raised on non-toxic plants, captive bred hornworms are fine.[16])

Horse Chestnut (*Aesculus hippocastanum*, all parts)

Horsetail Reed (*Equisetum*)

Hosta (*Hosta* genus, Plantain Lilies)

Hyacinth (*Hyacinthus orientalis*)

Hydrangea (*Hydrangea* genus)

Hydrogenated and Partially-Hydrogenated Oil

Indian Poke (*Veratrum viride*)

Iodized Salt (Table Salt)

Iris (*Iris* genus)

Iron Ammonium Citrate

Ivy (*Hedera,* ivy of any kind. Many ivys contain toxic properties when ingested. Conduct additional research based on specific variety.)

Jerusalem Cherry (*Solanum pseudocapsicum*, Nightshade family)

Jicama - skin, stem, seeds, leaves (*Pachyrhizus erosus*)

Jimsonweed (*Datura stramonium, Datura* genus)

Juniper (*Juniperus* genus)

Kalanchöe (*Kalanchöe* genus)

Lantana (*Lantana* genus)

Larkspur (*Delphinium* genus)

Laurels (*Kalmia latifolia,* also *Prunus* genus varieties)

- food additive | - natural insect repellent or insecticide

Lavender (*Lavandula* genus)

Leeks (*Allium ampeloprasum, porrum*)

Lemon (sour citrus varieties are generally unpopular)

Lemon Balm (*Melissa officinalis*)

Lemongrass (*Cymbopogon*)

Lichen (*Letharia and Vulpicida* species, see Appendix B)

Lily (*Lilium* genus, *Liliaceae* family)

Lily of the Valley (*Convallaria majalis*)

Lily of the Valley Bush (*Pieris japonica*)

Lime (sour citrus varieties are generally unpopular)

Lobelia (*Lobelia cardinalis, Lobelia* genus)

Lucky Bamboo (*Dracaena sanderiana*)

Lupine (*Lupinus* genus)

Manchineel Tree (*Hippomane mancinella*, Beach Apple, also spelled "manchioneel", "manchineal", "mancinella")

Mango - seeds, leaves, wood (*Mangifera indica*)

Marijuana (*Cannabis* varieties with THC content)

Marsh Marigold (*Caltha palustris*)

Mayweed (*Matricaria* genus)

Mescal (*Agave parryi*)

Microcrystalline Cellulose/MCC

Milkweed (*Asclepias* genus)

Mimosa Tree - seed pods (*Albizia julibrissin*, Persian Silk Tree)

Mistletoe (*Viscum album*)

Mold (in general, but especially in a closed environment, toxic species vary)

Monkshood (*Aconitum* genus)

Morning Glory (*Ipomoea violacea, carnea*)

Mother-in-Law's Tongue (*Sanseveria* genus)

Mountain Laurel (*Kalmia latifolia*)

Mums (*Chrysanthemum* species, *Asteraceae* family, source of pyrethrum/pyrethrin)

Mushrooms (those not identified for safe human consumption, toxic species vary)

Mustard Plant (*Brassica*)

Nandina (*Nandina* species, Heavenly Bamboo)

Narcissus (*Narcissus* genus)

Nectacot - seeds, stems, leaves, wood (hybrid of two *Prunus* species - nectarine and apricot)

Nectarine - seeds, stems, leaves, wood (*Prunus persica*)

Nightshade Family (*Solanum/Solanaceae*. While this family includes the potato, tomato, pepper, and eggplant, most plants in this family contain poisonous alkaloids. In general, all parts of the plants are considered toxic.)

Oleander (*Nerium oleander*)

Onion (*Allium cepa*)

Oregano (*Origanum vulgare,* blossoms are safe)

Oxeye Daisy (*Leucanthemum vulgare*)

Papaya - seeds (*Carica papaya*, Papaw)

Parsley - seeds (*Petroselinum crispum*)

Peace Lily (*Spathiphyllum* genus, contains insoluble calcium oxalate crystals)

Peach - seeds, stems, leaves, wood (*Prunus persica*)

Peacotum - seeds, stems, leaves, wood (hybrid of three *Prunus* species - peach, apricot, and plum)

Pear - seeds, stems, leaves, wood (*Pyrus* genus)

- food additive | - natural insect repellent or insecticide

Pencil Tree Cactus (*Euphorbia tirucalli*)

Pennyroyal (*Mentha pulegium*)

Peony (*Paeonia* genus)

Pepper - leaves, plant (*Capsicum*, Nightshade family)

Pepper, Ground (from peppercorns, the spice)

Peppercorns, all colors (*Piperaceae*, includes ground pepper, black pepper, source of piperine)

Peppermint (*Mentha piperita*)

Periwinkle Myrtle (*Vinca* species)

Persian Violet (*Cyclamen* genus)

Peyote (*Lophophora williamsii*)

Philodendron (*Philodendron* genus, contains insoluble calcium oxalate crystals)

Pine (*Pinus* genus)

Plantain Lily (*Hosta* genus)

Plum - seeds, stems, leaves, wood (*Prunus domestica*)

Pluots / Plumcots - seeds, stems, leaves, wood (hybrid of two *Prunus* species - plums and apricots, also called Aprium or Apriplums)

Poinsettia (*Euphorbia pulcherrima*)

Poison Hemlock (*Conium maculatum*)

Poison Ivy (*Toxicodendron radicans*)

Poison Oak (*Toxicodendron diversilobum*)

Poison Sumac (*Toxicodendron vernix*)

Pokeberry / Pokeweed (*Phytolacca* genus)

Polysorbate 80/P80

Poppy (*Papaver* genus)

Potato - sprouts/eyes, leaves, plant, green tubers/root (*Solanum tuberosum*, Nightshade family)

Pothos (*Epipremnum aureum*, contains insoluble calcium oxalate crystals)

Prickly Juniper (*Juniperus oxycedrus*)

Pride of China (*Koelreuteria paniculata*)

Privet (*Ligustrum* genus)

Prunus genus (This genus includes apricot, sweet almond, cherry, nectarine, peach, and plum. The fruit of these trees is edible, but everything else – seeds/pits, stems, leaves, bark, wood – contains cyanide-inducing glycosides and is considered poisonous to many species. In general, all parts of other Prunus plants are best avoided.)

Prussiate of Soda

Queen Anne's Lace (*Daucus carota*)

Ragworts (*Senecio* genus)

Ramps (*Allium tricoccum*)

Rapeseed / Rapeseed Oil (*Brassica napus*)

Red Emerald (*Philodendron*)

Red Maple - leaves (*Acer rubrum*, unidentified toxin affecting horses)

Redwood (*Sequoia sempervirens*)

Rhododendron (*Rhododendron* species)

Rhubarb - leaves (*Rheum rhaponticum*)

Rosary Pea (*Abrus precatorius*)

Rose - stems (*Rosa* genus, possible puncture hazard)

Rosemary (blossoms are safe)

Russian Thistle (*Salsola* genus)

Sago Palm (*Cycas revoluta*)

Salt (the generic word "salt")

Sanseveria (*Sanseveria* genus)

- food additive | - natural insect repellent or insecticide

Scallions (*Allium cepa*)

Scarlet Pimpernel (*Anagallis arvensis*)

Schefflera (*Schefflera* genus, Umbrella Plant, contains insoluble calcium oxalate crystals)

Scotch Broom (*Cytisus scoparius*)

Seasonings (the generic word "seasonings")

Senecio (*Senecio* genus, Ragworts)

Shallots (*Allium ascalonicum*)

Shasta Daisy (*Leucanthemum, Asteraceae* family)

Silicon Dioxide

Snake Plant (*Sanseveria* genus)

Snakeroots (*Ageratina* genus, *Asteraceae* family)

Sneezeweed (*Helenium* genus, an *Echinacea*/Coneflower look-alike)

Sneezewort (*Achillea ptarmica,* also called Sneezeweed)

Sodium Caseinate

Sodium Chloride

Solanaceae/Solanum Family (Most plants in this Nightshade family contain poisonous alkaloids. In general, all parts of the plants are considered toxic. See individual entries for eggplant, pepper, potato, and tomato plants.)

Soy Protein

Soy Protein Isolate

Soy Protein Concentrate

Spices (the generic word "spices")

Spurge (*Euphorbia* genus)

St. John's Wort (*Hypericum*, also called "Rose of Sharon")

Star Anise Fruit (*Illicium verum, I. anisatum*)

Stargazer Lily (*Lilium x Stargazer*)

Stearic Acid

Stock (the generic word "stock")

Suicide Tree (*Cerbera odollam*)

Sulfates / Sulphates

Sulfites / Sulphites

Sulfur Dioxide / Sulphur Dioxide

Sundew (*Drosera rotundifolia, Drosera* genus)

Sweet Almond - leaves, wood (*Prunus dulcis*)

Sweet Flag (*Acorus calamus*)

Sweet Melissa (*Melissa officinalis*)

Table Salt (Iodized Salt)

Tansy (*Tanacetum vulgare*)

Tarweed (*Amsinckia* genus)

Tea Tree (*Melaleuca alternifolia*)

Temple Bells (*Pieris japonica*)

Texas Mountain Laurel (*Sophora secundiflora*)

Textured Protein

Thorn Apple (*Datura stramonium*)

Thorns (possible puncture hazard)

Thyme (*Thymus vulgaris*, blossoms are safe)

Tiger Lily (*Lilium lancifolium*)

Tobacco (*Nicotiana* genus, Nightshade family)

Tomato - leaves, stems, plant, unripe fruit (*Solanum lycopersicum*, Nightshade family)

Toyon (*Heteromeles arbutifolia*, Christmas Berry)

Trillium (*Trillium* genus)

Trumpet Vine (*Campsis radicans*)

Tuba Root (*Derris Elliptica*)

Tulips (*Tulipa* genus)

Tumbleweed (*Salsola kali, S. tragus*, Russian Thistle)

Ultra-Pasteurized anything

Umbrella Plant/Tree (*Schefflera* genus, contains insoluble calcium oxalate crystals)

Venus Flytrap (*Dionaea muscipula*)

Verbena (*Verbena* genus)

Vinca (*Vinca* genus)

Walnut, Black (*Juglans nigra*)

Walnut, English - bark, wood (*Juglans regia*)

Water Hemlock (*Cicuta maculata*)

Whey Protein

Whey Protein Concentrate

Whey Protein Isolate

White Snakeroot (*Ageratina altissima*)

Wild Angelica (*Angelica sylvestris*)

Windflowers (*Anemone* genus)

Wisteria (*Wisteria* genus)

Wolfbane (*Aconitum* genus)

Wormwood (*Artemisia absinthium*)

Xanthan Gum

Xylitol (Birch Sugar, synthetic sweetener)

Yarrow (*Achillea millefolium*)

Yeast Extract

Yeast Nutrient

Yellow Jasmine (*Gelsemium sempervirens*)

Yerba Santa (*Eriodictyon californica*)

Yew (*Taxus baccata, Taxaceae*)

Yuca - root, plant (*Manihot esculenta*)

Yucca - root, leaves (*Yucca* genus, leaves - possible puncture hazard)

Zeolite

Zinc Oxide

---

[10] Bansal, Sheel et al. "Typha (Cattail) Invasion in North American Wetlands: Biology, Regional Problems, Impacts, Ecosystem Services, and Management."

[11] Temkin, Alexis et al. "Tests Find Hormone-Disrupting Fungicides on Most Citrus Fruit Samples."

[12] Osweiler, Gary D. "Slaframine Toxicosis."

[13] Kooyers, Nicholas J. et al. "Aridity shapes cyanogenesis cline evolution in white clover (Trifolium repens L.)"

[14] Deane, "Goldenrod Glorified."

[15] USDA Agricultural Research Service. "Rayless Goldenrod (Haplopappus heterophyllus)"

[16] Ivana and Bryce. "Crickets, roaches, and worms, OH my!"

Notes

- food additive | - natural insect repellent or insecticide

Bad Additives

What follows are ingredients commonly added to commercial and processed foods. Though there is no actual scientific proof that some of these additives are harmful specifically to hermit crabs, this list was created in an effort to reduce potential harm. The key to supplementing a diet for hermit crabs with manufactured products is informed label reading.

Anti-Caking Agents (i.e. silicon dioxide, calcium silicate, iron ammonium citrate, prussiate of soda)

Artificial Color, Flavoring, Sweeteners

Ascorbyl Palmitate

Aspartame

Autolyzed Yeast

Barley Malt

Benzoates

BHA (Butylated hydroxyanisole)

BHT (Butylated hydroxytoluene)

Birch Sugar (Xylitol, synthetic sweetener)

Bouillon / Broth (the generic word "broth")

By Products (the generic word "by product")

Calcium Caseinate / Calcium Silicate

Copper Sulfate

Emulsifiers (i.e. xanthan gum, canola oil, carboxymethylcellulose/CMC, polysorbate 80/P80, microcrystalline cellulose/MCC)

Enzymes and Enzyme Modified, anything

Ethoxyquin

Fermented, anything

Flavor(s) and Flavoring(s), Flavor Enhancers

Foaming Agents

Food Coloring

Gelatin

Glutamate

Glutamic Acid

High Fructose Corn Syrup

Hydrogenated Oil

Hydrolyzed Corn Gluten

Hydrolyzed Protein (any protein that is hydrolyzed)

Magnesium Oxide

Magnesium Stearate

Malt Extract and Flavoring

Maltodextrin

Menadione

Monopotassium Glutamate

Monosodium Glutamate (MSG)

Natural Beef Flavoring

Natural Chicken Flavoring

Natural Pork Flavoring

Partially-Hydrogenated Oil

Pepper, Black

Preservatives

Propylene Glycol

Protease and Protease Enzymes

Protein Fortified, anything

Prussiate of Soda (sodium ferrocyanide)

Salt, Iodized (Table Salt)

Seasonings (the generic word "seasonings")

Sodium Caseinate

Sodium Chloride

Soy Protein (includes Concentrate and Isolate)

Spices (the generic word "spices")

Stearic Acid

Stock (the generic word "stock")

Sulfates / Sulphates

Sulfites / Sulphites

Sulfur Dioxide / Sulphur Dioxide

Textured Protein

Ultra-Pasteurized, anything

Whey Protein (includes Concentrate and Isolate)

Xylitol (Birch Sugar, synthetic sweetener)

Yeast Extract

Yeast Nutrient

Zeolite

Zinc Oxide

"When in doubt - leave it out."

Sources:

Crab, Julia (2005). "Adulterants & Additives in hermit crab food." *The Crab Street Journal*. https://crabstreetjournal.org/blog/2015/09/19/adulterants-additives-in-hermit-crab-food/

Victoria State Government, Better Health Channel. "Food Additives". https://www.betterhealth.vic.gov.au/health/ConditionsAndTreatments/food-additives

Notes

Appendix A : Moss Varieties

⋙ When foraged, most – if not all – moss species are generally considered safe. See "Foraged Finds" for additional sourcing and preparation information.

⋙ Avoid moss that is labeled "preserved" and/or appears to be dyed as is often found with floral and hobby supplies.

The following species underwent additional research by Stacy Griffith of the Land Hermit Crab Owners Society and *The Crab Street Journal* to provide the botanical names of a few "safe" varieties.

American Tree Moss (*Climacium americanum*)

Baby Tooth Moss (*Plagiomnium cuspidatum*)

Big Shaggy-Moss (*Rhytidiadelphus triquetrus*)

Cushion Moss (*Leucobryum glaucum*)

Dwarf Haircap Moss (*Polytrichum juniperinum*)

Feather Moss (*Hypnum imponens*)

Fern Moss (*Thuidium delicatulum*)

Fire Moss (*Ceratodon purpureus*)

Glittering Wood Moss (*Hylocomium splendens*)

Haircap Moss, Common (*Polytrichum commune*)

Heath Star Moss (*Campylopus introflexus*)

Hoary Fringe-Moss (*Racomitrium canescens*)

Iceland Moss (*Cetraria islandica*, a lichen)

Juniper Moss (*Polytrichum juniperinum*)

Mood Moss (*Dicranum scoparium*)

Oak Moss (*Evernia prunastri*, a lichen)

Peat Moss, Common (*Sphagnum centrale*)

Plume Moss (*Ptilium crista-castrensis*)

Ribbed Bog Moss (*Aulacomnium palustre*)

Rigid Beard Moss (*Didymodon rigidulus*)

Sheet Moss (*Hypnum cupressiforme*)

Shiny Seductive Moss (*Entodon seductrix*)

Smoothcap Moss, Common (*Atrichum undulatum*)

Spanish Moss (*Tillandsia Usneoides,* epiphytic air plant, not really a moss)

Sphagnum Moss (*Sphagnum cymbilifolium*)

Spoon-Leaved Moss (*Bryoandersonia illecebra*)

Springy Turf Moss (*Rhytidiadelphus squarrosus*)

Star Moss (*Tortula ruralis*)

Tamarisk Moss, Common (*Thuidium tamariscinum*)

Tousled Treasure (*Callicladium haldanianum*)

Warnstorf's Peat Moss (*Sphagnum warnstorfii*)

Notes

Appendix B : Lichen Varieties

While many species of lichen are generally considered safe – a few are not.

⋙ All lichen that may be consumed should be soaked in several changes of water as leaching reduces the acid level and bitterness.[17]

⋙ For a more extensive photographic listing of lichen species by geographical region, visit: http://bit.ly/GeoLichen (https://lichenportal.org/cnalh/projects/index.php?pid=519)

The following varieties underwent additional research by Stacy Griffith of the Land Hermit Crab Owners Society and *The Crab Street Journal* to provide the botanical names of some "safe" and "unsafe" varieties.

Safe Lichen

Beard Lichen (*Usnea* genus)

British Soldiers (*Cladonia cristatella*)

Cup Lichen (*Cladonia* genus)

Dog Lichen (*Peltigera canina*)

Iceland Moss (*Cetraria islandica*, a lichen)

Manna (*Lecanora*)

Oakmoss / Oak Moss (*Evernia prunastri,* a lichen)

Parmelia (*Parmelia* genus)

Reindeer Lichen (*Cladonia* genus)

Roccella (*Roccella* genus)

Rock Tripe (*Umbilicaria*)

Tree Lungwort (*Lobaria pulmonaria*)

Verrucaria (*Verrucaria* genus)

Yellow Scales (*Xanthoria parietina*)

---

[17] Deane. "Usnea: Food and Pharmacy Lichen".

Notes

Unsafe Lichen

⋙ The genus *Letharia* and the genus *Vulpicida* are generally found in the Northern Hemisphere, in mountain forests (usually coniferous) – frequently at medium to high elevations, and often in cold, shaded sites. They are typically tolerant of snow burial.[18]

⋙ Both genus categories contain vulpinic acid that functions to discourage herbivore eating and has been shown to be relatively toxic to carnivorous mammals, as well as insects and mollusks.

⋙ All of the lichens below tend to be a bright yellow, yellow-green, or chartreuse in color.[18]

Letharia genus - "Wolf Lichen"

Letharia vulpina

Letharia columbiana

Vulpicida genus

V. canadensis Räsänen J.-E.Mattsson & M.J.Lai

V. juniperinus L. J.-E.Mattsson & M.J.Lai

V. pinastri Scop. J.-E.Mattsson & M.J.Lai

V. tilesii Ach. J.-E.Mattsson & M.J.Lai

V. tubulosus Schaer. J.-E.Mattsson & M.J.Lai

V. viridis Schwein. J.-E.Mattsson & M.J.Lai

[18] Consortium of North American Lichen Herbaria, https://lichenportal.org; information compiled from individual species pages.

Notes

Appendix C : Natural Plant Defenses

A full discussion of all of the plant-produced toxins in existence exceeds the scope and intention of this guide, but a few brief explanations may clarify some decisions made regarding some of the items in the preceding pages. Additional reading references (with regard to humans) and the sources used have been included for those that are curious and would like to conduct further research.

So, why do so many plants contain toxins? Simply put – plants just want to live, too. Over the years, many plants have evolved or been cultivated to develop chemical defense mechanisms to protect themselves from being decimated by things that eat them. The parts of a plant which are often used as food sources include the leaves, buds, stems, roots, fruit, roots/tubers, and seeds/nuts – and the toxins can reside in all or only a few of these parts.[19]

For some types of natural toxins, certain processing treatments and cooking can result in destroying the toxic substance or reducing its toxicity. Other toxins can remain unchanged even after processing and, in these cases, special care should be exercised in selecting the food plants, limiting the amount of intake, or eliminating them as options altogether.[19]

To read more about a variety of natural plant toxins in general, visit the source:

"Natural Toxins in Food Plants" »» http://bit.ly/NaturalToxins (https://www.cfs.gov.hk/english/programme/programme_rafs/programme_rafs_fc_01_17_report.html)

Lectins

⋙ Lectins are contained in all food to some degree with an estimated 30% of the foods commonly eaten in the United States containing significant amounts.[20]

⋙ Beans/legumes (*Fabaceae* family) such as kidney beans, soybeans, and peanuts contain the most plant lectins, followed by grains and plants in the Nightshade family.[20]

⋙ Lectins resist being broken down in the gut and are stable in acidic environments. Some animal and cell studies indicate that active lectins can interfere with the absorption of minerals, especially calcium, iron, phosphorus, and zinc.[21]

⋙ Mature, hard, dry legumes from typically inedible pods have higher concentrations of lectins than soft, fresh legumes like peas and green beans.[22]

⋙ Lectins are easily deactivated through cooking.[20] As such, beans/legumes in the "safe" list are marked with a symbol indicating they should be cooked first.

For more in-depth information about lectins in plants, visit the sources:

"Everything You Need to Know About Dietary Lectins" »» http://bit.ly/DietaryLectins
(https://www.healthline.com/nutrition/dietary-lectins)

"Lectins." »» http://bit.ly/MoreLectins
(https://www.hsph.harvard.edu/nutritionsource/anti-nutrients/lectins/)

"The Green Bean Controversy." »» http://bit.ly/BeansPeas
(https://www.thepaleomom.com/green-beans-peas/)

Cyanogenic Glycosides

⋙ Cyanide-inducing compounds known as cyanogenic glycosides are naturally present in many plants used as food, including apples (seeds), peaches (pits), apricots (pits), and bamboo shoots.[23]

⋙ In simplest terms, the plant stores the cyanide in an inactive form in two "compartments" within its cells. The cyanide does not become active until the two "compartments" are mixed through chewing or crushing.[24]

⋙ Cyanide essentially prevents cells from using oxygen, causing asphyxiation at the molecular level. It is effective against most life forms.[24]

⋙ A few studies have shown that some herbivores and invertebrates have developed ways to avoid being poisoned through modified behavior, either by varying the amount eaten or by simply being deterred by the bitter taste. Other studies indicate that some arthropods may have developed cyanide detoxification enzymes.[25] At this time, no study has been found that definitively states that land hermit crabs specifically are equipped to deal with the effects of cyanogenic glycosides.

⋙ In no-choice feeding experiments, when no other food is available in the habitat, herbivores may eat a larger amount of cyanide-defended plants leading to intoxication or death.[25]

⋙ As scary as cyanide poisoning may sound, cyanide is water soluble and relatively easy to eliminate. Generally, all that has to be done is to crush the plant and thoroughly wash the mash.[24] As it is not heat stable, boiling/cooking is also an effective method.

⋙ Even easier – simply do not offer the plant parts, like the leaves, stems, or pits in the *Prunus* family, that contain cyanogenic glycosides.[24]

⋙ Plants with particularly high amounts of cyanide (like cassava/yuca root and bamboo shoots) require specific, additional, often labor intensive preparation methods [24] that extend beyond the scope of this guide and these items have therefore been left on the "unsafe" list.

To learn more about cyanide in plants and herbivore adaptations to cyanide, visit the sources:

"A Review of Cyanogenic Glycosides in Edible Plants" »» http://bit.ly/CGPlants
(https://www.intechopen.com/books/toxicology-new-aspects-to-this-scientific-conundrum/a-review-of-cyanogenic-glycosides-in-edible-plants)

"Beware the smell of bitter almonds: Why do many food plants contain cyanide?" »» http://bit.ly/PlantsCyanide
(https://phys.org/news/2010-07-beware-bitter-almonds-food-cyanide.html)

"Herbivore Adaptations to Plant Cyanide Defenses" »» http://bit.ly/HerbivoresAdapt
(https://www.intechopen.com/books/herbivores/herbivore-adaptations-to-plant-cyanide-defenses)

Alkaloids » Glycoalkaloids » Solanine

⋙ Toxic alkaloids produced by plants can act as natural pesticides and are bitter in taste to deter herbivores (including humans) from eating them.[26]

⋙ Alkaloids are a very large group of compounds with a wide range of activities – some undesirable, some desirable, and some yet unknown – on both animals and humans. Some of these effects are anti-bacterial, anti-inflammatory, analgesic, hypnotic, psychotropic, amongst others. Well known plant derived alkaloids include morphine, strychnine, quinine, atropine, caffeine, ephedrine, and nicotine.[26]

⋙ Alkaloids, specifically the glycoalkaloid "solanine", are found in all members of the *Solanaceae/Solanum* (Nightshade) family, particularly in the leaves, stems, unripe fruit, and root of the few with edible fruits.[27, 28]

⋙ Potatoes, tomatoes, peppers, and eggplants are all common Nightshades and rich sources of nutrients. Many spices safe for hermit crabs come from these plants, like cayenne pepper, crushed red pepper, chili powder, and paprika.[27]

⋙ The solanine glycoalkaloid is normally present in all potato tubers in small amounts but is concentrated in the skin and in the eye/sprout regions. Levels are highest in green potatoes and can reach very high levels in the sprouts.[28, 29]

⋙ Solanine is not decreased by washing, soaking, or cooking*, making avoidance of the parts of the plant containing the glycoalkaloid the only safe course of

* boiling, microwaving, baking; Deep frying was more effective in tests with potatoes.[28]

action. For example, peel potatoes, do not offer green potatoes, green tomatoes, or the leaves/stems of any plant in the Nightshade family, and feed these foods in moderation as part of a varied diet.[28, 29]

⋙ Typically, insects eat only one or a small range of plant species and have developed ways of dealing with the toxic compounds in those particular plants. Some of these insects have evolved to a point where plant toxins form part of their own defenses, storing the poisons to ward off predators [30] – like the hornworm that feeds primarily on the leaves of Nightshades (or the monarch butterfly caterpillar that feeds primarily on milkweed). Hence, do not feed wild caught hornworms.

To read more about plant alkaloids and the edible members of the Nightshade family, visit the sources:

"Introductory Chapter: Alkaloids - Their Importance in Nature and for Human Life" »» http://bit.ly/AlkaloidNature (https://www.intechopen.com/books/alkaloids-their-importance-in-nature-and-human-life/introductory-chapter-alkaloids-their-importance-in-nature-and-for-human-life)

"Are Nightshades Bad for You?" »» http://bit.ly/NightVegs (https://www.healthline.com/nutrition/nightshade-vegetables)

"A Review of Occurrence of Glycoalkaloids in Potato and Potato Products" »» http://bit.ly/TaterReview (https://www.foodandnutritionjournal.org/volume4number3/a-review-of-occurrence-of-glycoalkaloids-in-potato-and-potato-products/)

"Should you be afraid of green potatoes?" »» http://bit.ly/GreenTaters (https://www.eatortoss.com/single-post/2016/03/26/the-truth-about-green-potatoes)

"Australian Native Poisonous Plants." »»
http://bit.ly/AussiePlants
(http://anpsa.org.au/APOL7/sep97-4.html)

---

[19] Centre for Food Safety. "Natural Toxins in Food Plants."

[20] Leech, Joe. "Everything You Need to Know About Dietary Lectins."

[21] Harvard T.H.Chan School of Public Health. "Lectins."

[22] Ballantyne, Dr. Sarah. "The Green Bean Controversy."

[23] Bolarinwa, Islamiyat Folashade et al. "A Review of Cyanogenic Glycosides in Edible Plants."

[24] Lutz, Diana. "Beware the smell of bitter almonds: Why do many food plants contain cyanide?"

[25] van Ohlen, M., Herfurth, A.-M., Wittstock, U. (2017). "Herbivore Adaptations to Plant Cyanide Defenses."

[26] Kurek, Joanna. "Introductory Chapter: Alkaloids - Their Importance in Nature and for Human Life."

[27] Pearson, Keith (2020). "Are Nightshades Bad for You?"

[28] Omayio D. G, Abong G. O, Okoth M. W. "A Review of Occurrence of Glycoalkaloids in Potato and Potato Products."

[29] Eat or Toss. "Should you be afraid of green potatoes?"

[30] "McKenzie, Dr. Ross. "Australian Native Poisonous Plants."

Notes

References
and Works Consulted

Many of the items compiled in this pocket guide were obtained from lists citing The All-Natural Hermit Crab Sourcebook (Arenella and Michaelson, 2004) as their originating source and expanded on by experienced hermit crab keepers over the years — primarily those updated, maintained, and distributed online by the Land Hermit Crab Owners Society and *The Crab Street Journal*.

These lists – as well as items added during the creation of this guide – were cross referenced with other safe and toxic lists, studies, and articles published on the web as noted below.

As research evolves with regard to the effect of various ingredients specifically on land hermit crabs, the items in the preceding pages may change after publication. For the latest "safe" and "unsafe" food and foraging lists, please visit *The Crab Street Journal* online (crabstreetjournal.org) or the official Land Hermit Crab Owners Society Facebook Group (facebook.com/groups/landhermitcrabowners).

Arenella, Stacey and Michaelson, Summer (2004). The All-Natural Hermit Crab Sourcebook, p. 30-35. ISBN: 0-9755887-0-2.

ASPCA. "Catsear." https://www.aspca.org/pet-care/animal-poison-control/toxic-and-non-toxic-plants/catsear, date accessed: 4.16.2021.

ASPCA. "Golden Bells." https://www.aspca.org/pet-care/animal-poison-control/toxic-and-non-toxic-plants/golden-bells, date accessed: 3.13.2021.

ASPCA. "Milkweed". https://www.aspca.org/pet-care/animal-poison-control/toxic-and-non-toxic-plants/milkweed, date accessed: 4.22.2021.

ASPCA. "Pampas Grass". https://www.aspca.org/pet-care/animal-poison-control/toxic-and-non-toxic-plants/pampas-grass, date accessed: 2.18.2021.

ASPCA. "Poisonous Plants. Toxic and Non-Toxic Plants List." https://www.aspca.org/pet-care/animal-poison-control/toxic-and-non-toxic-plants. Used to cross reference existing lists and ingredients found in all-natural hermit crab supplier foods.

Ballantyne, Dr. Sarah (2016). "The Green Bean Controversy." *The Paleo Mom*. https://www.thepaleomom.com/green-beans-peas/, date accessed: 2.18.2021.

Bamboo Plants HQ. "Is bamboo edible or is it toxic?" https://bambooplantshq.com/is-bamboo-edible-or-is-it-toxic/, date accessed: 3.18.2021.

Bansai, Sheel et al. (2109) "Typha (Cattail) Invasion in North American Wetlands: Biology, Regional Problems, Impacts, Ecosystem Services, and Management." *Wetlands*. Volume 39, pps. 645-684.

Bantam.Earth. "Vivarium Moss & Moss-Like Plants." https://bantam.earth/vivarium-moss/, date accessed: 4.21.2021.

Biomin. "Vibrio in shrimp aquaculture - Causes, symptoms and prevention measures." https://www.biomin.net/species/aquaculture/vibriosis/, date accessed: 4.16.2021.

Birdsafe.com. "Safe and Dangerous Woods." http://www.birdsafe.com/woods.htm, date accessed: 3.6.2021.

Bolarinwa, Islamiyat Folashade et al. (2016) "A Review of Cyanogenic Glycosides in Edible Plants." https://www.intechopen.com/books/toxicology-new-aspects-to-this-scientific-conundrum/a-review-of-cyanogenic-glycosides-in-edible-plants, date accessed: 4.21.2021.

Bonnie Plants. "How to Dry Your Harvest." https://bonnieplants.com/gardening/how-to-dry-your-harvest/, date accessed: 5.3.2021.

CAB International, Invasive Species Compendium. "Rhizophora mangle (red mangrove)". https://www.cabi.org/isc/datasheet/47509#touses, date accessed: 2.18.2021.

Campbell, Kerie (2005). "Going Natural Beginner's List." *The Crab Street Journal*. https://crabstreetjournal.org/blog/2015/04/07/going-natural-beginners-list/, date accessed: 2.18.2021.

Carey, Dennis and Avent, Tony (January 2010). "Buddleia davidii: The Butterfly Bush." *Plant Delights Nursery, Inc.* https://www.plantdelights.com/blogs/articles/butterfly-bush-buddleia-davidii-plant-buddleja, date accessed: 3.31.2021.

Centre for Food Safety, The Government of the Hong Kong Special Administrative Region. (March 2007) "Natural Toxins in Food Plants." https://www.cfs.gov.hk/english/programme/programme_rafs/programme_rafs_fc_01_17_report.html, date accessed: 4.21.2021.

Colorado State University - Guide to Poisonous Plants. "Red Maple." https://csuvth.colostate.edu/poisonous_plants/Plants/Details/87, date accessed: 5.13.2021.

Consortium of North American Lichen Herbaria, https://lichenportal.org, date accessed: 4.22.2021 - used to cross reference the lichen species of the genus *Letharia* and the genus *Vulpicida* with regard to coloration and regional distribution.

Crab, Julia (2005). "Adulterants & Additives in hermit crab food." *The Crab Street Journal*. https://crabstreetjournal.org/blog/2015/09/19/adulterants-additives-in-hermit-crab-food/, date accessed: 1.21.2021.

Crab, Julia (2005). "Safe Edible Flowers for Hermit Crabs." *The Crab Street Journal*. https://crabstreetjournal.org/blog/2015/09/19/edible-flowers-for-hermit-crabs/, date accessed: 2.18.2021.

Crush, J. R., Caradus, J. R. (1995) "Cyanogenesis potential and iodine concentrationin white clover (Trifolium repens L.) cultivars." *New Zealand Journal of Agricultural Research*. Vol. 38, Issue 3, pps. 309-316.

Deane. "Century Plant: Edible Agave Americana." *Eat the Weeds and other things, too*. http://www.eattheweeds.com/century-plant/, date accessed: 5.13.2021.

Deane. "Eastern Red Bud: Pea Pods Tree." *Eat the Weeds and other things, too*. http://www.eattheweeds.com/eastern-red-bud-pea-pods-on-a-tree, date accessed, 3.21.2021.

Deane. "Goldenrod Glorified." *Eat the Weeds and other things, too*. http://www.eattheweeds.com/solidago-odora-liberty-tea-2/, date accessed: 5.1.2021.

Deane. "Hydrilla." *Eat the Weeds and other things, too*. http://www.eattheweeds.com/hydrilla/, date accessed, 4.16.2021.

Deane. "Indian, Mock Strawberry." *Eat the Weeds and other things, too*. http://www.eattheweeds.com/potentilla-indica-mistaken-identity-2/, date accessed: 3.21.2021.

Deane. "Maple Manna." *Eat the Weeds and other things, too.* http://www.eattheweeds.com/?s=maple, date accessed: 5.13.2021.

Deane. "Reindeer Moss." *Eat the Weeds and other things, too.* http://www.eattheweeds.com/tag/cladonia-cristatella/, date accessed: 5.12.2021.

Deane. "Usnea: Food and Pharmacy Lichen." *Eat the Weeds and other things, too*. http://www.eattheweeds.com/usnea-food-and-pharmacy-lichen/, date accessed: 5.12.2021.

Deane. "Violets' Virtues." *Eat the Weeds and other things, too.* http://www.eattheweeds.com/viola-affinis-floridas-sweet-violet-2/, date accessed: 5.19.2021.

Dyer, Mary H. "Does Anise Repel Bugs: Information On Natural Anise Pest Control." *Gardening Know How.* https://www.gardeningknowhow.com/edible/herbs/anise/natural-anise-pest-control.htm, date accessed: 4.18.2021.

Eat or Toss. "Should you be afraid of green potatoes?" https://www.eatortoss.com/single-post/2016/03/26/the-truth-about-green-potatoes, date accessed: 4.21.2021.

Emmerich, Robert et al. (1993) "Toxicity and Antifeedant Activity of Lichen Compounds Against the Polyphagous Herbivorous Insect Spodoptera Littoralis." *Phytochemistry*, Vol 33, No 6. pp. 1389-1394.

Farnen, Johnny O. "Wood for Use in Vivaria." *Caudata Culture*. https://www.caudata.org/cc/articles/wood.shtml, date accessed: 3.6.2021.

Garden Gate Magazine. "Look out for these plants toxic to fish." https://www.gardengatemagazine.com/articles/flowers-plants/plant-guide/poisonous_plants/, date accessed: 3.5.2021.

Gardner, Zoë and McGuffin, Michael (2013). American Herbal Products Association's Botanical Safety Handbook, Second Edition, p. 523-526. ISBN: 978-1-4665-1694-6.

Gardners' World.com. "Arbutus unedo." https://www.gardenersworld.com/plants/arbutus-unedo/, date accessed: 3.6.2021.

Griffith, Stacy. "Organic Explained." *LHCOS Facebook Group*. https://www.facebook.com/notes/land-hermit-crab-owners-society/organic-explained/1531278340369850/, date accessed: 2.21.2021.

Growables Grow Florida Edibles. "Custard Apple - Annona reticulata." https://www.growables.org/information/TropicalFruit/annonareticulata-new.htm, date accessed: 3.10.2021.

Harvard T.H.Chan School of Public Health. "Lectins." https://www.hsph.harvard.edu/nutritionsource/anti-nutrients/lectins/, date accessed: 4.22.2021.

Ivana and Bryce. "Crickets, roaches, and worms, OH my!" *Illinois State University.* https://vetmed.illinois.edu/wel/crickets-roaches-and-worms-oh-my/, date accessed: 3.7.2021.

Jacques, Erica. "Flax Meat & Cyanide." *Livestrong*. https://www.livestrong.com/article/538409-flax-meal-cyanide/, date accessed: 4.21.2021.

Julson, Erica (2018). "Can You Eat Kiwi Skin?" *Healthline.* https://www.healthline.com/nutrition/eating-kiwi-skin, date accessed: 7.3.2021.

Karriker, Kent. "Jewelweed (Impatiens capensis)." *USDA - U.S. Forest Service*. https://www.fs.fed.us/wildflowers/plant-of-the-week/impatiens_capensis.shtml, date accessed: 3.30.2021.

Kilamanjaro's Hermits. "Harvesting". http://kilimanjaroshermits.blogspot.com/p/harvestables.html, date accessed: 2.6.2021.

Kooyers, Nicholas J. et al. (2014) "Aridity shapes cyanogenesis cline evolution in white clover (Trifolium repens L.)" *Molecular Ecology. Vol.* 23, Issue 5, pps. 1053–1070.

Kurek, Joanna (2019). "Introductory Chapter: Alkaloids - Their Importance in Nature and for Human Life." https://www.intechopen.com/books/alkaloids-their-importance-in-nature-and-human-life/introductory-chapter-alkaloids-their-importance-in-nature-and-for-human-life, date accessed: 4.22.2021.

Lady Bird Johnson Wildflower Center. "Ruellia humilis." https://www.wildflower.org/plants/result.php?id_plant=ruhu, date accessed: 3.30.2021.

Lama, Siddhi Camila (November 2018). "Is It Safe to Eat Bean Sprouts Raw?" *Livestrong*. https://www.livestrong.com/article/456815-can-you-eat-bean-sprouts-raw/, date accessed 7.3.2021.

Lamont, Carrie (2014). "Berries of the Vaccinium Family." *Dave's Garden*. https://davesgarden.com/guides/articles/view/5215, date accessed: 4.23.2021.

Lawry, James D. "Vulpinic and Pinastric Acids as Lichen Antiherbivore Compounds: Contrary Evidence." *The Bryologist*, Vol. 86, No. 4 (Winter, 1983), p. 365.

Leech, Joe (2019). "Everything You Need to Know About Dietary Lectins." *Healthline*. https://www.healthline.com/nutrition/dietary-lectins, date accessed: 4.21.2021.

Lindinger, Dr. Michael. (August 2019). "Ground flaxseed – How much can we and our companion animals safely eat?" *Nutraceutical Alliance*. https://www.nutraceuticalalliance.ca/post/ground-flaxseed-how-much-can-we-and-our-companion-animals-safely-eat, date accessed: 4.21.2021.

Lutz, Diana (2010). "Beware the smell of bitter almonds: Why do many food plants contain cyanide?" *Phys.org*. https://phys.org/news/2010-07-beware-bitter-almonds-food-cyanide.html, date accessed: 3.26.2021.

M.D. Vaden. "Bird perches, toys. Safe & harmful perch wood." https://mdvaden.com/bird_page.shtml, date accessed: 3.6.2021.

McKenzie, Dr. Ross. "Australian Native Poisonous Plants." http://anpsa.org.au/APOL7/sep97-4.html, date accessed: 3.10.2021.

McPartland, John M. (1997). "Cannabis as repellent and pesticide." *Journal of the International Hemp Association*. https://druglibrary.net/olsen/HEMP/IHA/jiha4210.html, date accessed: 3.28.2021.

Modern Pest Services (2016). " Natural Pest Control: 4 Flowers For Your Garden." https://www.modernpest.com/blog/natural-pest-control-garden/, date accessed: 4.17.2021.

Nash, Thomas H. (1996). "Lichen Biology". *Cambridge University Press*. p. 179.

Natesan, Sivakumar, and Gopal, Selvakumar. "Effect of Different Carbon and Nitrogen Sources on the Production of Carotenoid Pigments by Phaffia rhodozyma." *ResearchGate*. https://www.researchgate.net/publication/325719659_Effect_of_Different_Carbon_and_Nitrogen_Sources_on_the_Production_of_Carotenoid_Pigments_by_Phaffia_rhodozyma, date accessed: 3.12.2021.

National Center for Biotechnology Information. "Veronica Plants—Drifting from Farm to Traditional Healing, Food Application, and Phytopharmacology." https://www.ncbi.nlm.nih.gov/pmc/articles/PMC6651156/, date accessed: 3.13.2021.

National Center for Home Food Preservation. "Drying", https://nchfp.uga.edu/how/dry/pack_store.html, date accessed: 2.18.2021.

Nick, Jean (2018). "Are Stone Fruit Seeds Poisonous?" *Good Housekeeping*. https://www.goodhousekeeping.com/health/diet-nutrition/a20705824/are-stone-fruit-seeds-poisonous/, date accessed: 5.6.2021.

Norms Farms. " Are Elderberry Bushes Poisonous?" https://normsfarms.com/blogs/growing-and-harvesting-elderberry/are-elderberry-bushes-poisonous, date accessed: 4.21.2021.

North Carolina Plant Toolbox, Extension Gardner. "Impatiens balsamina." https://plants.ces.ncsu.edu/plants/impatiens-balsamina/, date accessed: 3.31.2021.

Omayio D. G, Abong G. O, Okoth M. W. (2016). "A Review of Occurrence of Glycoalkaloids in Potato and Potato Products." *Current Research in Nutrition and Food Science*. https://www.foodandnutritionjournal.org/volume4number3/a-review-of-occurrence-of-glycoalkaloids-in-potato-and-potato-products/, date accessed: 4.21.2021.

Oregon Health Authority. "Safe Eating of Shellfish." https://www.oregon.gov/oha/ph/HealthyEnvironments/Recreation/Documents/Shellfish-safety.pdf

Osweiler, Gary D. "Slaframine Toxicosis." *Merck Manual, Veterinary Manual*. https://www.merckvetmanual.com/toxicology/mycotoxicoses/slaframine-toxicosis, date accessed: 4.21.2021.

Pearson, Keith (2020). "Are Nightshades Bad for You?" *Healthline*. https://www.healthline.com/nutrition/nightshade-vegetables, date accessed: 4.21.2021.

Peary, Warren and Peavy, William. "Natural Toxins in Sprouted Seeds: Separating Myth from Reality." *Sentrex Systems Manufacturing*. https://sproutnet.com/natural-toxins-in-sprouted-seeds/, date accessed: 4.21.2021.

Petal Republic. "Ultimate Guide to Coreopsis Flower Meaning, Origins, Uses, Gifting, and How to Grow at Home." https://www.petalrepublic.com/coreopsis-flowers/, date accessed: 5.1.2021.

Petruzzello, Melissa. "7 of the World's Deadliest Plants." *Britannica*. https://www.britannica.com/list/7-of-the-worlds-deadliest-plants, date accessed: 5.6.2021.

Plants Database - USDA. "Cornus florida L. flowering dogwood." https://plants.usda.gov/plantguide/pdf/pg_cofl2.pdf, date accessed: 3.6.2021.

Plants For A Future. https://pfaf.org. Used to cross reference existing lists and ingredients found in all-natural hermit crab supplier foods.

Plants For A Future. "Albizia julibrissin - Durazz." / Mimosa. https://pfaf.org/user/Plant.aspx?LatinName=Albizia+julibrissin, date accessed: 2.18.2021.

Plants For A Future. "Alnus glutinosa" / European Alder, Common Alder. https://pfaf.org/user/plant.aspx?latinname=Alnus+glutinosa, date accessed: 2.21.2021.

Plants For A Future. "Alnus incana" / Grey Alder. https://pfaf.org/user/Plant.aspx?LatinName=Alnus+incana, date accessed: 2.21.2021.

Plants For A Future. "Alnus rhombifolia" / White Alder. https://pfaf.org/user/Plant.aspx?LatinName=Alnus+rhombifolia, date accessed: 2.21.2021.

Plants For A Future. "Alnus rubra" / Red Alder. https://pfaf.org/user/Plant.aspx?LatinName=Alnus+rubra, date accessed: 2.21.2021.

Plants For A Future. " Annona muricata - L." / Soursop. https://pfaf.org/user/Plant.aspx?LatinName=Annona+muricata, date accessed: 2.18.2021.

Plants For A Future. " Camellia japonica - L." / Camellia. https://pfaf.org/User/Plant.aspx?LatinName=Camellia+japonica, date accessed: 2.18.2021.

Plants For A Future. "Cercis canadensis - L." / Redbud. https://pfaf.org/user/Plant.aspx?LatinName=Cercis+canadensis, date accessed: 3.21.2021.

Plants For A Future. "Chaenomeles speciosa - (Sweet.)Nakai." / Flowering Quince.https://pfaf.org/user/Plant.aspx?LatinName=Chaenomeles+speciosa, date accessed: 3.30.2021.

Plants For A Future. "Claytonia virginica - L." / Spring Beauty. https://pfaf.org/user/plant.aspx?LatinName=Claytonia+virginica, date accessed: 3.30.2021.

Plants For A Future. "Cortaderia selloana" / Pampas Grass. https://pfaf.org/user/Plant.aspx?LatinName=Cortaderia+selloa na, date accessed: 2.18.2021.

Plants For A Future. "Daucus carota L." / Queen Anne's Lace. https://pfaf.org/user/Plant.aspx?LatinName=Daucus+carota, date accessed: 4.21.2021.

Plants For A Future. "Edible Ornamental Plants." https://pfaf.org/user/cmspage.aspx?pageid=78, date accessed: 3.30.2021.

Plants For A Future. "Fagus grandifolia - Ehrh." / American Beech. https://pfaf.org/USER/Plant.aspx?LatinName=Fagus+grandifolia, date accessed: 5.13.2021.

Plants For A Future. "Forsythia x intermedia - Zabel." / Forsythia. https://pfaf.org/user/Plant.aspx?LatinName=Forsythia+x+intermed ia, date accessed: 3.13.2021.

Plants For A Future. "Hippophae rhamnoides - L." / Sea Buckthorn. https://pfaf.org/user/Plant.aspx?LatinName=Hippophae+rhamnoi des, date accessed: 2.18.2021.

Plants For A Future. "Linum usitatissimum - L." / Flax. https://pfaf.org/user/Plant.aspx?LatinName=Linum+usitatissimum, date accessed: 4.21.2021.

Plants For A Future. "Nelumbo nuciferaa - Gaertn." / Sacred Water Lotus. https://pfaf.org/user/Plant.aspx?LatinName=Nelumbo+nucif era, date accessed: 4.16.2021.

Plants For A Future. "Persea americana - Mill." / Avocado. https://pfaf.org/user/Plant.aspx?LatinName=Persea+americana, date accessed: 2.18.2021.

Plants For A Future. "Phlox paniculata - L." https://pfaf.org/user/Plant.aspx?LatinName=Phlox+paniculata, date accessed: 4.28.2021.

Plants For A Future. "Pieris japonica - (Thunb.)D.Don." / Lily of the Valley Bush. https://pfaf.org/User/Plant.aspx?LatinName=Pieris+japonica, date accessed: 4.16.2021.

Plants For A Future. "Pueraria montana lobata - (Willd.) Sanjappa & Pradeep." / Kudzu Vine. https://pfaf.org/user/Plant.aspx?LatinNa me=Pueraria+montana+lobata, date accessed: 4.16.2021.

Plants For A Future. "Rheum rhaponticum - L." / Rhubarb. https://pfaf.org/user/Plant.aspx?LatinName=Rheum+rhaponticum, date accessed: 2.18.2021.

Plants For A Future. "Robinia pseudoacacia - L." / Black Locust. https://pfaf.org/user/plant.aspx?latinname=Robinia+pseudoacacia, date accessed: 3.30.2021.

Plants For A Future. "Rudbeckia hirta - L." / Black Eyed Susan. https://pfaf.org/user/Plant.aspx?LatinName=Rudbeckia+hirta, date accessed: 4.17.2021.

Plants For A Future. "Trifolium pratense - L." / Red Clover. https://pfaf.org/user/Plant.aspx?LatinName=trifolium+pratense, date accessed: 4.21.2021.

Plants For A Future. "Trifolium repens - L." / White Clover. https://pfaf.org/user/plant.aspx?LatinName=Trifolium+repens, date accessed: 4.21.2021.

Plants For A Future. "Tropaeolum majus - L." / Nasturtium. https://pfaf.org/user/plant.aspx?LatinName=Tropaeolum+majus, date accessed: 4.18.2021.

Plants For A Future. "Yucca baccata - Torr." / Yucca. https://pfaf.org/user/Plant.aspx?LatinName=Yucca+baccata, date accessed: 3.30.2021.

Platt, Steven G. et al. "Canebrake fauna revisited: additional records of species diversity in a critically endangered ecosystem." *The Journal of the American Bamboo Society*, Vol 26. https://bamboo.org/_uploads/pdfs/BSCv26.pdf, date accessed: 3.6.2021.

Pond Informer. "List of Plants Toxic to Pond Fish (Common Poison Species)." https://pondinformer.com/plants-toxic-to-pond-fish/, date accessed: 3.21.2021.

Ready Store. "What is the Shelf-Life of an Open Can?" https://www.thereadystore.com/blog/shelf-life-open-10, date accessed: 4.16.2021.

Ruttan, Ally and Lortie, Christopher E. (2015). "A systematic review of the attractant-decoy and repellent-plant hypotheses: do plants with heterospecific neighbours escape herbivory?" *Journal of Plant Ecology*, Volume 8, Number 4, pps. 337-346.

Said Musallam Al Alawi; Hossain, Mohammad Amzad; Ahmed, A.Abusham. "Antimicrobial and cytotoxic comparative study of different extracts of Omani and Sudanese Gum acacia." *ScienceDirect*. https://www.sciencedirect.com/science/article/pii/S2314853517300951, date acccessed: 3.6.2021.

Salehi, Bahare, et al. "Lamium Plants—A Comprehensive Review on Health Benefits and Biological Activities." *National Center for Biotechnology Information*, May 2019. https://www.ncbi.nlm.nih.gov/pmc/articles/PMC6571824/, date accessed: 3.13.2021.

Salzet, M. Stefano, G.B. (February 1, 2002). "The endocannabinoid system in invertebrates." *Elsevoir Science Ltd.* https://www.plefa.com/article/S0952-3278(01)90347-3/pdf

Southern Living. "Best and Worst Flowers to Plant for a Pet-Friendly Garden". https://www.southernliving.com/garden/flowers/pet-friendly-plants, date accessed: 2.6.2021.

Southern Research Station - USDA. "Cornus florida L.; Flowering Dogwood." https://www.srs.fs.usda.gov/pubs/misc/ag_654/volume_2/cornus/florida.htm, date accessed, 3.10.2021.

Spritzler, Franziska (2017). "Oxalate (Oxalic Acid): Good or Bad?" *Healthline*. https://www.healthline.com/nutrition/oxalate-good-or-bad, date accessed: 2.18.2021.

Tavares, Wagner De Souza et al. (October 2011). "Insecticide activity of piperine: toxicity to eggs of Spodoptera frugiperda (Lepidoptera: Noctuidae) and Diatraea saccharalis (Lepidoptera: Pyralidae) and phytotoxicity on several vegetables." *Journal of Medicinal Plant Research. Volume* 5(21), pp. 5301-5306.

Temkin, Alexis et al. (March 2021). " Tests Find Hormone-Disrupting Fungicides on Most Citrus Fruit Samples." *Shopper's Guide to Pesticides in Produce*. https://www.ewg.org/foodnews/citrus.php, date accessed: 7.3.2021.

Texas A&M AgriLife Extension. "Landscape IPM, Botanical Insecticides." https://landscapeipm.tamu.edu/types-of-pest-control/chemical-control/organic/botanical/, date accessed, 7.3.2021.

The Crab Street Journal. "FAQ What foods are good and bad for hermit crabs?" https://crabstreetjournal.org/blog/2012/10/16/faq-what-foods-are-good-and-bad-for-hermit-crabs/, date accessed: 1.31.2021.

The Crab Street Journal. "Foods for Hermit Crabs." https://docs.google.com/document/d/113toruv4u7NJxPYdM8-xVXZ7W4duiC54EvKqrh33-pY/edit, date accessed: 1.31.2021.

The Crab Street Journal. "Hermit Crab Feeding Guide." https://crabstreetjournal.org/download/hermit-crab-feeding-guide/, downloaded: 1.31.2021.

The Crab Street Journal. "Hermit Crab Food Foraging List." https://crabstreetjournal.org/blog/2016/05/12/hermit-crab-food-foraging-list/, date accessed: 1.31.2021.

The Crab Street Journal. "Hermit Crab Food Foraging List, PDF." https://crabstreetjournal.org/download/Foraging-List-Final-Rev4-2019.pdf, date accessed: 1.31.2021.

The Crab Street Journal. "Hermit Crab Nutritional Table." https://crabstreetjournal.org/download/Download-Print-Share/Hermit-Crab-Nutrional-Table-2019.pdf, date accessed: 1.31.2021.

The Crab Street Journal. "What's for dinner? A hermit crab food guide!". https://crabstreetjournal.org/blog/2016/04/22/hermit-crab-food-guide/, date accessed: 1.31.2021.

The Crab Street Journal. "FAQ What foods are good and bad for hermit crabs?" https://crabstreetjournal.org/blog/2012/10/16/faq-what-foods-are-good-and-bad-for-hermit-crabs/,
date accessed: 1.31.2021.

The Tortoise Table. https://www.thetortoisetable.org.uk/
Used to cross reference existing safe/unsafe lists.

The Tortoise Table. "Coneflower." https://www.thetortoisetable.org.uk/plant-database/viewplants/?plant=101&c=5#.YI71KN0pBhE, date accessed: 5.2.2021.

The Tortoise Table. "Sneezeweed." https://www.thetortoisetable.org.uk/plant-database/viewplants/?plant=604#.YI71o90pBhF, date accessed: 5.2.2021.

The Tortoise Table. "Sneezewort." https://www.thetortoisetable.org.uk/plant-database/viewplants/?plant=798#.YI74tt0pBhF, date accessed: 5.2.2021.

Tilton, Lois (April 22, 2009). "Beans! Beans! The Poisonous Fruit!" *Dave's Garden*. https://davesgarden.com/guides/articles/view/2385,
date accessed, 2.13.2021.

University of California Safe and Poisonous Garden Plants. "Safe Plants (by common name)." https://ucanr.edu/sites/poisonous_safe_plants/Safe_Plants_by_Common_Name/, date accessed: 3.6.2021.

USDA Agricultural Research Service. "Rayless Goldenrod (Haplopappus heterophyllus)" https://www.ars.usda.gov/pacific-west-area/logan-ut/poisonous-plant-research/docs/rayless-goldenrod-haplopappus-heterophyllus/, date accessed: 5.1.2021.

van Ohlen, M., Herfurth, A.-M., Wittstock, U. (2017). "Herbivore Adaptations to Plant Cyanide Defenses." https://www.intechopen.com/books/herbivores/herbivore-adaptations-to-plant-cyanide-defenses, date accessed: 4.22.2021.

Victoria State Government, Better Health Channel. "Food Additives". https://www.betterhealth.vic.gov.au/health/ConditionsAndTreatments/food-additives, date accessed: 2.18.2021.

Vila, Bob. "10 Plants to Grow for a Pest-Proof Yard." https://www.bobvila.com/slideshow/10-plants-to-grow-for-a-pest-proof-yard-49121, date accessed: 4.18.2021.

What's Cooking America. "Edible Flowers Chart." https://whatscookingamerica.net/EdibleFlowers/EdibleFlowersMain.htm, date accessed: 2.13.2021.

Wholesome Children. "Elderberries: Healthy or Toxic?" https://wholesomechildren.com/using-fresh-raw-elderberries-safely/, date accessed: 4.21.2021.

Wilson, Rhonda (September 2007). "The Planted Tank: From Pond to Aquarium." *Tropical Fish Hobbyist Magazine*. https://www.tfhmagazine.com/articles/aquatic-plants/from-pond-to-aquarium, date accessed: 4.1.2021.

World Chelonian Trust. "Plants That Poison". http://www.chelonia.org/articles/plantsthatpoison.htm, date accessed: 2.2.2021- used to cross reference existing lists and ingredients found in all-natural hermit crab supplier foods.

Zanchett, Giliane and Oliveira-Filho, Eduardo C (2013). "Cyanobacteria and Cyanotoxins: From Impacts on Aquatic Ecosystems and Human Health to Anticarcinogenic Effects." *Toxins* Volume 10, Number 10. pps. 1890-1917.

Notes

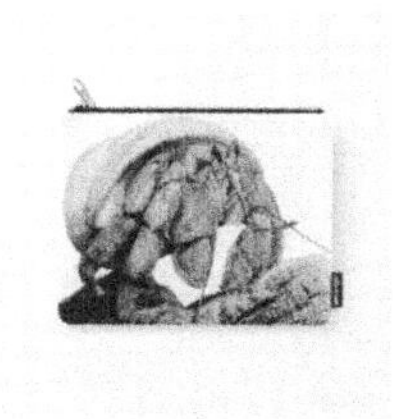
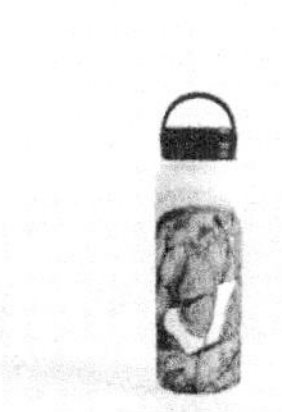
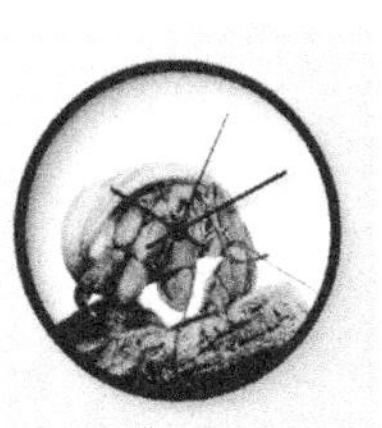
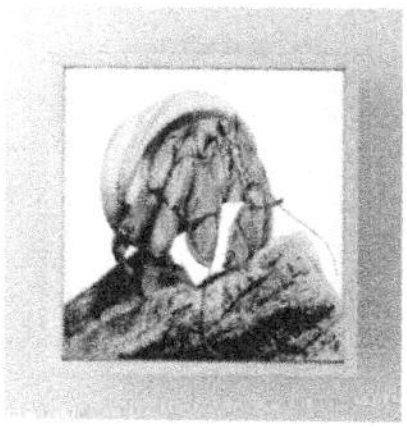

Made in the USA
Monee, IL
13 September 2026

63137524R00066